TOTAL HEALTH

George Green

Total Health

* * * * * * * *

A search for healthy living

* * * * * * * * *

George Green

Total Health

Feel free to contact the author at

geogreen100@gmail.com

Address

George Green
8930 S Painter Ave #105
Whittier, CA 90602

Total Health

DISCLAIMER

Disclaimer: [Any of the information contained in these articles is for informational and educational purposes only, it is not intended to cure or heal any disease. No medical claim is made regarding any of this information. The author has studied natural medicine for many years in search of better health for himself; however he does not claim to be neither a medical doctor nor any type of health practitioner. Every person is responsible to consult with a doctor before undertaking any of the advice given in these articles. The articles written here are the sole opinion of the author based on his years of study of nutrition and health issues. The author does not guarantee or promise any kind of results from following this advice. The author is not liable in any way shape or form for any negative results from any advice given here. The author opinion shall be considered that only his opinion, based upon the constitution guaranteed freedom of speech]

I am sorry I had to give this disclaimer, but I have attacked very powerful industries and interests in this book and despite our guaranteed freedom of speech; I fear that one of those interests might want to silence my voice for speaking the truth by filing some frivolous lawsuit. Unfortunately we live in a litigious society, and any person could be sued or be taken to court on just about anything, even for speaking the truth.

Also a person given health or nutritional advice could be prosecuted under the charge of practicing medicine without a license, even if the information is correct and beneficial. Unfortunately the medical establishment principal interest is not to the health and well being of people, but their own financial well being. Anything that threatens the financial interest of the medical establishment is attacked regardless of how truthful or beneficial it might be.

Much of what I write about goes against the interests of very powerful industries that have billions of dollars at their disposal and would just love to silence my voice. I just do not have the resources to defend myself in court nor the desire to spend the rest of my life being dragged into court. Without a disclaimer I could be sued under the flimsiest excuse.

Now that I have explained the reason for this disclaimer, let me say that I have researched deeply all the information given here and I am confident that the information I give is mostly correct. I have researched book after book in order to glean the best advice from the top health experts. Of course all of these articles are written in my own style and are just my personal opinion. I may be wrong in some parts, but I am willing to correct those parts in the near future, as soon as I find credible research that contradicts my opinions.

A lot of what I have written might go against the advice given by some nutritionists and other health advisors, but having researched carefully the pros and cons of different ideas and theories I have decided to stick to what I felt was the best way to follow to achieve total health.

George Green

I have tried to keep my writing simple I have not tried to confuse the issues by getting too technical. I am not writing for nutritional experts but for the common person. That is why I have purposely avoided talking about saturated fats, unsaturated fats, trans-fats, polyunsaturated fats, or talk about sucrose, and all the other nutritional terms.

I could have just given a list of don't and do's about nutrition and health, but then you would not understand the reasoning behind the advice that I give. By taking the time to explain each topic, in more detail, hopefully I will be able to convince you to adopt some of my recommendations.

I am fully aware that some people will dismiss my writings without even considering them, but I am also sure that there will be others who will listen, and understand that I am trying to teach the values and principles of total health.

Sincerely

A simple voice crying out in the wilderness

INTRODUCTION

Your health is extremely important, for your health is the most important possession you have. I know because I lost my health by years of careless living and ignorance. After I had a heart attack I realized that I was so sick that I would die soon, I then decided to prolong my life for as long as possible. I happen to be quite fond of living and not in a hurry to leave this world.

I have always been a reader, but I had not been interested in health issues. Well after my heart attack, I quickly became interested. I begun reading everything I could to get back my health. I slowly began to make changes in my life, well better late than never. Slowly I begun to recuperate and get better, I made lots of notes on my research on health. After a few years of research, I had made so many notes; that I then decided to write a book from all my research.

I had to learn from experience that having health is very important, living in misery and pain is definitely not a good place to be in. Thankfully all my pain and misery has gone away, but not because I kicked the bucket, but because I took the actions needed to get back my health. Yes it is possible to live a good life even when dealing with a disease, but it becomes an added life burden.

Many people when they lose their health, they also lose all hope, and even become suicidal. That is because nobody wants to live in pain and discomfort for the rest of their lives. Also many do not want to be a burden to their family. Being sick brings a whole new set of problems into anyone's life. I understand them for I too had thoughts of suicide, so I could be out of my misery and pain and did not want to be a charge to my family. When I was suffering I sincerely regretted my past mistakes and the lifestyle I had led, but that did not take away the suffering, I had to take action to stop the suffering.

Some people think that they cannot take the action needed to change their destructive lifestyle, well when it is your life in the line, believe me you will have enough motivation to change your lifestyle. You have to, because the only other option is to continue in the downward path of destruction. Of course some changes are easier than other to make, so if you want to be healthy start with the small steps and then go on to the bigger steps.

With all that said, let us continue talking about your health. Your health consists of your physical and mental health. Your whole body needs to be healthy. People who achieve success in life tend to be those who have a healthy lifestyle and purposely take care of their body and mind. You need to educate yourself and learn about your health, for no one else cares more about you than you.

Do not let Hollywood and the advertising media fool you into buying harmful products and items. You should only buy those things that are good and healthful for you, not what slick advertisers want you to buy and consume. You need to protect you health by shunning the unhealthy products and substances displayed in the media.

Our modern diet is a horrible diet. We eat the wrong foods and we eat too much of them. We eat foods too rich in the wrong substances; our prosperity is killing us. We need to eat a better diet, but most of us just can't sacrifice a little food today to have good health tomorrow. Simplicity and moderation are not welcomed words now days.

If our diet was not bad enough, let us not talk about our lifestyle. It is a lifestyle of no restraint. We party way too hard and sleep erratically. We spend hours staring at a TV or computer burning out our eye sockets. All electrical products emit radiation, and eventually this excessive radiation will have an effect and it will not be a good one.

Let us not get even mention about our lack of physical exercise. We spend hours and hours at the office sitting in a chair, and then we get home and sit for hours on the sofa. Is it any wonder we get flabby and fat. Fat is definitely a strong contributor to many grievous diseases.

Let us also not forget about our mental health. We suffer from excessive stress due to a constant barrage of bad news that only serves to alarm us and make us fearful and worried. We love to get scared or excited with horror or adventure movies. This entertainment raises our adrenaline yet we do not spend it on anything but keep it inside.

Many people do not want to hear about being healthy. They shut their ears to the messages of healthy living; that is until they get sick. When we do something about our health it is usually the wrong action. We go on bad diets, take horrible drugs, go into dangerous surgery, or some other fads that only make our health problems worse.

Table of Contents

PART I: THE BAD

JUST SAY NO

You have probably heard the message of just say no a million times. But why do so many people use hard drugs? Simple reason, because it makes them feel good, like someone once said about trying drugs "Don't try them, you'll like them". But what about legal drugs? A drug is a drug whether it is legal or not. There are many different types of drugs but they have one thing in common, they are all bad for your body and mind.

It is important to remember that drugs and chemical substances are illegal with the penalties being severe. When it comes down to it no laws can really stop those that are bent on breaking them. The choice to use drugs is really up to you. It is an issue of personal freedom; however you must remember that these substances will adversely affect your body and your mind.

HARD DRUGS: There is a very good reason why hard drugs are illegal. They are extremely harmful to your body and mind, and some of the damage is permanent. Once you get on them kiss your life and your future goodbye for it is very hard to get off them, and even after you manage to kick them the health damage is for life.

CHEMICALS: Chemicals are just not something you should inhale or put in your body in any way or shape. They were created for industrial use, and you are not a machine. You can not put in your body something designed for a machine.

NATURAL DRUGS: Come on let us not kid ourselves, just because something is natural does not mean you should eat it. Poison is natural; will you drink the poison of a snake, or a scorpion? Nature has drugs for natural purposes not necessarily for humans to eat.

MARIHUANA: This is the most common of the illegal drugs. Despite its illegality it is widely available. It relaxes the mind and stimulates the appetite. The fact that it isn't as destructive as the hard drugs does not make it a harmless diversion. There is definitely brain damage resulting from using marijuana.

MEDICAL DRUGS: Those are developed for the treatment of some disease, there is a good reason they are only prescribed by doctors. Many of the hard drugs were at one time used as medical drugs, until they showed up their true nature.

It is kind of hard to understand why some people would use a drug that will destroy them just so they can be considered "cool" or sophisticated. Drugs fads come and go, but not before leaving a path of destruction.

Healing from drug abuse is not easy. The drugs may eventually clear completely from your system, but the damaged caused may remain for a lifetime, also the craving for the drugs may remain for the rest of your life. There are many treatments geared toward helping the drug addicted recover, but avoid those that use drugs to cure drugs.

There is absolutely nothing healthy about drugs. They will destroy you. If you use drugs you might as well kiss goodbye to your health, your mind, your money, your job, your freedom, your family and possibly your life.

UP IN SMOKE

What hasn't been said about the dangers of tobacco? Yet plenty of people still light up. Tobacco affects the body and mind, it gives a relaxing feeling and it is highly addictive. With all the bad publicity about smoking you would think that the tobacco industries would be bankrupt, but to the contrary. They are still raking in big money.

The tobacco industry is billions of dollars rich, they have an arsenal of lawyers at their disposal and are not afraid to use them. They have the money to hire the best advertising agencies in the world and pay the highest politicians in the land. And they are not afraid to take on the medical establishment either.

Tobacco is grown and processed specially to make it as highly addictive as possible. They have teams of scientists wholly dedicated to making sure that once a person becomes addicted to tobacco, they will stay addicted.

One of the biggest secrets of the tobacco industry is that they on purpose add substances that will make tobacco more addictive than what it is in its natural state. Of course they will keep all their ingredients a trade secret for they are allowed to do so. When people buy tobacco, they are getting many other chemicals along with it.

The fact that tobacco smoked, chewed or taken in any form causes cancer can not longer be denied. No filter or anything can make tobacco less dangerous. The tobacco industry fought for years to keep that fact from the public, but the evidence was so overwhelming that even with all their billions they just could not keep the truth from coming out.

Cancer is not the only harm that tobacco causes; it also contributes significantly to heart attacks and many other diseases. Many mental problems are enhanced by the use of tobacco or probably caused by it. And we shall not even mention the thousands of fires caused by cigarettes. The medical costs associated with tobacco use are astronomical.

The tobacco industries lose thousands of their customers per year, some quit, but the vast majority simply dies from using their products. So they have to find ways to lure new customers into their trap. They try to portrait tobacco as sophisticated, grown up, a macho thing to do, and any other positive image. They have the money to create slick enticing ads that will pull in new gullible customers. They target specifically the young with free giveaways and other enticements.

Tobacco stinks and it gets into the skin of the smokers and also into all its surroundings. Tobacco stink is so bad that many hotels will have separate rooms just for smokers. No matter what people use the stink penetrates deep into the fabrics and it is almost impossible to get rid of.

Many employers won't hire smokers, because of the stink, fire danger and high medical costs associated with smoking. Smokers not only kill themselves but they tend to kill those around them with second hand smoke.

FIREWATER

The Indians used to call alcohol firewater. And the name is appropriate for that is exactly what it does; it cooks your insides. The dangers of alcohol have been known from ancient times. Every holy book warns about the dangers of alcoholism.

The litany of what alcohol does to your body is long, but the best known is cirrhosis of the liver. Of course it also affects the mind, alcoholics tend to be mean people, and their mind is obsessed with alcohol. An alcoholic will resort to anything in order to sustain their habit; they will steal from their job, their family, their friends and strangers.

Of course the alcohol industries will never show you a filthy drunk in their commercials, but the gutter drunk is the end result of using their products. Of course they show you fun loving people enjoying their products. They seduce you with beautiful women in their commercials and they might occasionally throw in the line about drinking in moderation.

Of course the alcohol industry is a multi-billion dollar industry that protects its interests and will fight tooth and nail to have the right to peddle their poison to people. They will cite the evils of prohibition, and seek to discredit any of their critics. They will lavishly fund the politicians, and conduct sophisticated mass marketing campaigns.

They will loudly tout any study that proclaims alcohol to have some health benefits. Yes it is true that when used in moderation alcohol can be beneficial to the body, but many people don't know what moderation means. If you truly have a sense of moderation, then there is nothing wrong health-wise with drinking a cup of wine per day after lunch or dinner; it could actually be beneficial to your heart, remember just one cup per meal any more than that is not moderation.

Of course a couple of cups of wine per day is not what the alcohol barons want. They want you to chuck a whole bottle per day so that their profits will increase, your health be dammed. Do you think for any second that the alcohol barons give a hoot about your health? They simply want you to buy their products and use anything to encourage more people to drink their poison. Seriously folks, the few benefits that alcohol can give your body, are far outweighed by the harm that it could do.

Alcohol is a cultural thing, in many cultures alcohol is used in weddings and other festivities. However that is changing and more people are having festivities where no alcohol is served. If alcohol is being served and you are offered a cup you could graciously decline or accept it, but learn to stop at that cup.

Some people have good control of their drinking habits, and can make a can of beer last for an hour, while with others it wouldn't last a minute. Yes it is true that most drinkers do not become gutter drunks but some do, and plenty die before getting to that level.

Alcohol is addictive, so the more alcohol content is put into a drink the more addicted you become. That is why it is best to forget about drinking alcohol. It will destroy your liver, your mind and your health.

CHEMICAL DEATH

Humans are the only species that would purposely eat substances not meant to be eaten. I am talking about the chemicals that we put in our processed foods. It is plain madness and craziness to eat chemicals that will kill us, yet we modern people do it all the time. We supposed to be the most educated people of all the ages, but obviously we are ignorant of the dangers in those chemicals or we have been totally brainwashed.

Seriously folks we as a race must be real stupid to eat substances that are poisonous to our bodies. Wake up! The chemicals being put into processed foods arc killing us. I do not care what governmental agency has decreed that those chemicals are safe for us to eat, they can not convince others and me that they deadly, deadly, deadly.

First of all there are plenty of food chemicals that have been approved and then recalled when deadly and harmful effects have surfaced. Of course if the effects do not show up right away then the chemical is deemed safe. Come on people; who is fooling whom, the chemical and food industries pay tons of money to politicians. They have their own paid scientists and advertisers to babble whatever line is needed. And if that fails they have an army of lawyers ready to defend their chemical laced food products.

If you ever think of taking a food company to court because their harmful chemicals made you sick, you better have a billion dollars or a team of super lawyers, because the food industry has that and a whole lot more.

The food industry is in the business of making money, not in the business of providing nutritious or healthful foods. Any nutritional value in their food is just an incidental benefit not done on purpose. They put chemicals in the foods to make them last longer, taste better and make more money. Artificial flavors are put to fool our tongues into eating delicious garbage, but our bodies can not survive on garbage. Artificial colors are added to make junk food look pretty but who cares if poison looks pretty, it is still poison.

We can avoid most of those chemicals by avoiding canned or processed food, but that is not longer enough. Some grocers have now begun to tinker with natural foods. They have begun by adding a waxy substance to the apples in order to make them shiner. Excuse me but I am buying apples for their nutritional value, not because they shine pretty. I would not be surprised if the grocers one day came with a scheme to inject chemicals to the bananas in order to prevent them from going overripe. Unless we realize what is going on, the food industry would soon have us eating all our food with chemicals added, actually they almost have succeeded.

Let me repeat this again and again, chemicals are not food. I really don't know how long people could live on chemicals or what will be the long-term effects all those chemicals in our systems, but I can assure you it will not be pretty. If we keep on adding those dangerous and deadly chemicals to our foods, I can safely predict more cancer, diabetes, and other degenerative diseases coming our way in the near future.

Why do people keep on eating chemicals as food? Many do it because they don't think there are any options. Well there are options, you can return to eating natural foods and be safe. Yes, you can stop eating chemical loaded foods and eat natural organic foods. Throw those cans into the big can; that is where canned food really belongs in.

THE DAILY JOLT

In order to jumpstart their bodies many people resort to jolting their system with coffee. Coffee has a substance named caffeine that is what makes coffee stimulate the system. But caffeine is not confined to just coffee. This substance is also in chocolate, teas, guarana, kola nuts and it is the main ingredient in sodas and many candies.

Caffeine is not a harmless stimulating substance like some people think, or like the coffee industry would have you believed. It is a mild drug but do not let that fool you. It is a harmful stimulant that damages the nervous system and causes havoc with our sleep patterns. The list of health problems and diseases that caffeine creates or contributes to; is extensive. Yes it is also addictive and if you quit drinking caffeinated drinks you will get some withdrawal symptoms like headaches and low energy. I should know; for every time I have quite caffeine I usually go for a week with a headache.

THE DOUBLE WHAMMY: This is when caffeine is mixed with sugar. Not only do you get stimulation from the caffeine but you also get a sugar rush. This is a common and very harmful combination. It is like giving a one-two punch to the body system. And that is how most people take their caffeine.

COFFEE: Just by itself without any sugar, coffee is a big problem. It is not only the caffeine that is the problem but also the industrial process that is used to produce the coffee. Coffee is highly addictive and if taken daily will eventually sicken people.

SODAS: You might think that only the colas have caffeine, but you will be amazed to discover that other drinks also have caffeine in them. Just because they don't look black it doesn't mean they don't have caffeine, just read the label and you will find it.

ENERGY DRINKS: Besides being loaded with sugar and caffeine many energy drinks are also loaded with many other stimulating substances. Only time will tell what kind of horrible damage these new substances do to the body and mind.

CHOCOLATE: This is not the harmless drink that a family can share in a winter night or that lovers can send to their sweethearts on St. Valentine's Day. If you really love people you do not give them something that will hurt their health and chocolate definitely will hurt them. Chocolate has little caffeine, but it is loaded with sugar and fats. If you still want to have some chocolate then choose dark chocolate which has less sugar and fat than the other types.

TEA: Teas have been promoted as a healthful choice, and they are as long is they are not black teas for they do have much caffeine. Those advertised as decaffeinated still have about 4 percent caffeine, which is not a big amount but if the caffeine was removed by chemical process then avoid it. The best teas are the herbal ones without caffeine for only those could truly be classified as healthy.

The body can handle an occasional cup of coffee to stay alert, but problem is the daily use of coffee and the massive amounts used. The early cup of coffee will jolt people and wake them up, but once the caffeine wears out it will make them crash, so a little later they need their coffee break. That is why people go through the day drinking coffee, colas, and eating chocolate bars. They are simple addicted to caffeine. All this constant artificial jolting of the human body will eventually cause damage to the body and mind.

SWEET POISON

Refined sugar is not natural, it is a drug, yes it is; it is refined and purified just like other drugs are. It is also highly addictive; if you stop eating it you will suffer withdrawal symptoms like when quitting any other drug. Refined sugar tastes good and gives you a good feeling just like a drug would and it is harmful to your body just like a drug is. The massive amount of sugar in the modern diet contributes to a host of diseases. There are mountains of evidence pointing out the harmful effects of sugar and new research is adding more evidence to the problems of sugar.

Of course many people will think that attacking their beloved sugar is just not nice. After all sugar is sweet, makes them feel good and gives them lots of energy. Asking people to give up sugar is like asking drug addicts to give up dope. They are so used to sugar that they fail to recognize the dangers from sugar or if they know them they will dismiss them as of no importance. Many people need their sugar fix and no warnings or any amount of evidence will ever persuade them. They have purposely closed their ears and shut closed their eyes to all the evidence that points to the harm sugar does.

It is pointless to get into an argument about the chemical composition of sugar or that sugar is a simple carbohydrate, those points are irrelevant. Sugar is full of empty calories, nutritionally deficient and it is not a harmless stimulant; it is a deadly poison. Eating a diet composed of only sugar will definitely hurt you physically and mentally; it will even kill you, nothing sweet about that. It is a harmful substance that just happens to be legal and very popular. It contributes to a whole lot of diseases especially cancer and diabetes.

Refined sugar tastes good and makes us feel good. There is a very good reason for that;

the body needs sugar in order to function, but it does not need "Refined" sugar. The tongue itself has a part dedicated to the taste of sugar, but you need to get your sugar from fruits and other natural foods. Your body is not designed to handle refined sugar; it was designed to eat natural sweetness. Refined sugar is not natural it does not exist in nature; it is a man made product.

The main and most serious problem is that refined sugar is so purified and potent that it goes instantly into the body. That is what is called the "sugar rush". It feels great because the body gets an instant boost of energy. However the body was not made to handle such a load of sugar. The constant rush of sugar into the body every day tears down the body little by little and many people end up with cancer, diabetes and other diseases.

The body is made to handle natural sugar on an incremental basis, when you eat an apple; it is slowly dissolved and releases its sugar on a gradual basis. There is no "sugar rush" it is more like a "sugar walk". The sugar in fruits is healthy and it is called fructose. A great benefit of eating fruits; is that they also supply fiber, vitamins and other healthful substances. The body has no problem if you eat a whole bunch of apples, pears or bananas. Your stomach will be full long before you can get a "sugar rush".

The second problem with refined sugar is that the body becomes accustomed to it and wants more of it. A person might start by putting a spoon of sugar into his coffee, but eventually she will put two and then even go to three, or she might resort to having more cups during the day. People may start with the small soda but eventually end up drinking the big size. This incremental desire for sugar goes often unnoticed by the sugar addict.

The third problem is that if a person tries to quit eating sugar he is against two big obstacles. The first obstacle is that his body has become addicted to sugar and will fight any attempt to deny it its daily ration. The second obstacle is the market food aisles; it seems that every packaged food has some added sugar in it. The reason every product has sugar in it is simple; it is highly addictive and that makes people buy more of it.

The fourth problem is that any refined sugar not burned up with activity becomes fat and makes people gain weight. Why doesn't everybody develop diabetes then? For the simple reason that the body can withstand a lot of abuse. It takes a long time to wear down the body, that is why 90 percent of Type 2 Diabetic patients are over 40 and obese, it took years for the body to finally give up. Of course there are other contributing factors like genetics and a sedentary lifestyle.

The effects of sugar on children are well known. A heavy diet of sugary cereals will make them hyperactive. They have wild mood swings, with high periods of energy followed by periods of extreme exhaustion; that only a dose of sugar can relieve, then the whole cycle starts again. These kids don't need Ritalin; they are strung out on sugar.

The body is very resistant and could handle a small amount of refined sugar with no problem, but not the excessive amounts many feed it. Many people get to work and immediately get their coffee with sugar and some will even add a sugary donut. They will keep on eating sugary foods and drinks through the day. Just add all the sugar from the coffee, the sodas and the candy bars and you will see a big problem.

Of course the sugar industry denies their product causes any harm, they have billions of dollars at stake. But there is so much damming evidence that it is beginning to look like a replay of the tobacco industry which for years denied their products caused cancer. It is well proven that sugar makes people fat, and people will get sick physically and mentally in a diet of pure sugar. The evidence is all there for those who want to accept it.

Refined sugar was unknown in the ancient world. People used to sweeten their foods with honey. Diabetes was a rare disease. People still managed to live healthy lives without the need for sugar in their diets. Sugar is not needed in any foods, it is added to foods. Sugar adds a lot of empty calories, and it depletes the body of vitamins and minerals

Ancient skulls reveal few cavities even in old people, and toothpaste did not exist. For hundredths of years none of the foods in the market contained any sugar. When refined sugar became available it was an expensive commodity. Only those with money could afford to buy it. Diabetes was first labeled as a rich man's disease; it did not exist among the poor. The effects of sugar in causing many diseases became apparent after a while.

There is a whole lot more that could be said about the ill effects of sugar on human beings; history is replete with stories about the damage that the introduction of sugar has caused upon primitive cultures that didn't have refined sugar in their diets. People who don't use refined sugar in their diets suffer from fewer diseases; than those who use it.

THE TRUE AND BITTER FACT IS THAT REFINED SUGAR IS BAD, BAD, BAD.

A PINCH IS ENOUGH

Salt contains sodium, which is an essential ingredient for our bodies, without it we would definitely go mad and die. That is why nature provides it naturally in milk, eggs, vegetables and meats. There is nothing wrong with salt, except our excessive eating of it. We eat way too much salt, beyond what we normally need.

The body has an efficient mechanism for dealing with excess salt; it disposes of salt through our sweat and our urine. But the body can not handle the massive amounts of salt in our current diet without penalizing us. That is the reason why high blood pressure is such a prevalent disease in our society.

High blood pressure or hypertension leads to kidney failure, heart disease and other problems with your health. Many young kids are developing hypertension due to the massive amounts of salt in their diets. And many more will develop it along the way because the body can only take abuse for so long.

Sailors already know the dangers of too much salt. A good sailor would never drink a glass of seawater on purpose, because he knows that all that excessive salt would dehydrate him, and make it him thirstier. The end result of drinking seawater would result in madness and an excruciating death. Yet many people gladly will eat more salt than there is in a bucket of seawater.

We are supposed to eat an average of 5 grams of salt per day, of course some people need different amounts, it all depends on body chemistry and how active a person is, but the problem is that the majority of people eat three times that amount daily.

Of course an athletic person will definitely need more than 5 grams; that is why they take those sports drinks. Soldiers used to take salt tablets with them into battle, because the demands of battle drained their bodies of vital salts. Under extreme exercise, hot temperatures, stress and harsh conditions the body of course needs more salt.

If you work outdoors in the heat of the day make sure that you wear some hat, drink plenty of water. Watch out for signs of dehydration and if you feel tired then have a salty snack like a small bag of pretzels or some salted peanuts.

Never, never, never buy the salt sold in the stores, for it is the worst kind, and has been processed and refined with poisonous chemicals. Get your salt from a health food store and make sure that it is sea salt. The best salt comes from the sea, it has our needed sodium and it also contains many good minerals. Iodine is frequently added to salt to prevent gout; that is why it is better to buy iodized salt. If you live by the ocean you can even make your own salt. Some people make kosher salt, which is better to use in meats.

Not all salts are the same, depending on where the salt comes from; it will have different minerals and taste slightly different. Salt from marshes seems to have the most minerals. If you accidentally put too much salt in a meal throw in a potato which will absorb the excess salt. If you have dry meat, then soak it for a couple of hours to take away the excess salt. Just remember that when it comes to salt, a pinch is enough.

FAT EVERYWHERE

There is plenty of bad publicity about fat, so everyone is aware of that. However let me say that fat is good. You need to eat some fat in your diet in order for your body to function correctly. Fat is used in many body processes, and without fat in your system you will definitely die. However what your body certainly doesn't need is the massive amounts of fats in our daily diets. Get this in your head, fat is good, excessive fat is bad. You need a little fat, but you don't need gobs of fat.

Nature provides you with plenty of good fat; you do not need to add more to your foods. Plenty of natural foods have their own fat. Foods like avocados, olives, nuts and others produce their own fat. There is absolutely no need to avoid these natural foods. This is the healthy fat that nature intended for us to eat.

Of course we also get fat from the meat of animals but animal fat is not good at all for us. We need to avoid eating the fat of animals; that is why we to need to eat lean cuts of meat. That is the main problem with hamburgers and other processed meats. The fat is not taken out of the meats but is mixed in with the meat in the grinding. Greasy fat give the meat a good taste but it is like eating a delicious poison.

There are some steps you can take to cut down on the fat from animals. Eat those meats low in fat, things like fish, chicken or turkey. Eat little of those meats that are higher in fat like beef. Cut the fat out of the meat, you don't have to be fanatical about it, but do cut the biggest sections of fat, give them to your dog or cat or just throw it away. Do not eat the skin of the chicken; it is where most of the fat resides in the chicken, also make sure that you buy only ground meat with a low fat content of less than 15%.

When people eat excessive fat we all know it goes to the belly or bottom and it makes us fat. Fat makes us fat, it makes sense. But what most people don't know is that excessive fat also affects adversely the brain. Research has shown that too much fat affects the brain. A person who eats a fat rich diet is usually groggy after lunch. His mind has trouble concentrating on the job and even feels like falling asleep.

Should then people avoid all fatty foods? No. Do not avoid any foods that have natural fat in them already, what you need to do is to avoid adding more fat to them. There is absolutely nothing wrong with eating natural fats; that is why nature provided them to us, for our health, so go ahead and eat those nuts.

You also need to avoid eating all those fat laden chocolate candies, donuts, pork products and other fried and processed foods. They are overloaded with fat, which you really don't need at all. Most people fail to realize that a massive amount of fat is hidden in many products; the only way to find out is to read the ingredient's list. You will be amazed at the number of foods that contain excessive hidden fat.

The point is to have a balance of how much fat you put in and how much fat you are burning out through regular activities and exercise. It is perfectly ok to be about five pounds overweight. That is your body's reserve for an emergency. What you should be striving is to avoid having so much body fat that it becomes a health hazard to you.

WHITE DEATH

The bread that formerly was called the staff of life has now become the staff of death. How has this conversion been accomplished? Simply, by the modern means of processing. The bread that is on most people table has been stripped of its natural nutrients and goodness. It is now not only lifeless but has been turned into a disease producer. How can bread be deathly? Because most bread is now made with processed white flour.

Most people do not realize it but for centuries people ate brown bread and never developed any diseases from eating whole bread, it is only in the last 50 years that bread itself has become a cause of sickness.

But bread is not the only place where this white deathly powder hides. It is also used to make cookies, flour tortillas and many other products. It is often added to many other products as an additional ingredient. The reason is simple, white flour tastes good, but it is nutritional suicide.

Why is white flour deathly? Because of the way it is manufactured. The modern production of wheat is accomplished by using artificial fertilizers and pesticides. Even though the majority of these artificial poisons and ingredients remain in the ground a small amount does make it into the wheat product, and eventually will reach our table.

Later on when the wheat is gathered into modern barns more chemical gases or poisons are often pumped into them. This is done to prevent vermin infestation and mold from growing. The problem is that small traces of those poisons remain in the wheat and those small traces of poisons are then passed on to us.

Later on the wheat will be refined and be stripped of all natural vitamins and nutrients, and be turned into flour. This refinement is done in order to keep the wheat from spoiling and also makes it easier for transportation.

Then the wheat is put through a process that whitens it by using bleachers and other chemical process. White flour is not natural; it is made that way by using chemical bleachers that whiten the flour to a nice looking white color. The ancients ate plenty of bread but none of it was white. White flour is a modern invention and a deathly one.

The harmful effects of white flour run the gamut of the whole medical dictionary. They created allergies, worsen diabetes, and worsen many other diseases. The devastating health effects of white flour should enough to ban it from any table.

Not only that, but white flour has zero nutritional value. It is a bunch of empty calories that does not provide any nutrition; you might as well be eating a piece of cardboard. The claim of fortified bread made by the manufacturers is bogus. The bread manufacturers only restore a small portion of vitamins in the bread and to make matters worse those are synthetic vitamins, which are almost worthless to the body.

The simplest solution is to avoid all white flour and go back to eating whole-wheat flour, which is the ancient and healthy way to eat bread, cookies and other wheat products. Yes whole wheat goes rancid faster and does not taste as good as white bread, but after a while you get used to eating it and you get a healthier body.

THE OTHER WHITE MEAT

The one animal that should never be eaten is the pig; this includes any pig products too. This is an animal full of toxins and excessive fat. It also has a lot of bacteria and some parasites that will make people sick. I am quite positive that many of today's diseases and health problems come from eating pork meat.

Jews and Muslims have clearly understood the dangers of eating pork meat and have prohibited their people against it. There is nothing positive or good about pig meat. In Mexico I saw pigs running wild and they ate the most disgusting things imaginable. The reason pigs do that is because they are following what they were designed to do.

All the animals in nature have a purpose; the purpose of the pig is to be a sort of vacuum machine of nature. The pig eats the filth and rotting flesh of the dead animals. It is a way for nature to recycle fast its natural resources. Nature has so endowed the pig with a system that is able to eat what no other animal would.

The religious prohibition against eating the pig, which comes from the Bible, has never been explicitly declared null. When the first gentile converts came into the church it was decided that they could come in without having to observe the law like the Jewish converts. So the gentile Christians disregarded the Jewish laws without realizing that some of those laws had for centuries protected the Jewish nation from disease.

During the dark ages plagues and pestilence killed thousands of people in Europe, however the Jewish population escaped these diseases, this gave rise to accusations that the Jews had made deals with the devil. The Jewish escaped those diseases in part because of their rituals and because they abstained from eating pig meat.

I really don't have enough strong words to describe how dangerous and poisonous pig meat is. Just because people do not immediately drop on the spot they think that it is OK to eat pork. They fail to realize that the poison slowly but surely accumulates in their system, but eventually disease will come. When cancer or some other hideous disease strikes a person, that person often wonders why. I do not wonder, I do know that their eating habits created those diseases. The more people eat pork meat the greater their chances of dying young.

Of course the pork meat producers will deny and attack these statements, well what else would you expect from them, they are only protecting their source of income. No the pork producers are not evil people in any way; they are simple people who lack the knowledge or refuse to believe that their products are hurting people. If they want to keep on selling pig meat and people continue buying it, they have every right to do so. I just refuse to participate in my own destruction.

There is a ton of research that has been done on the subject of the effects of eating pig meat. But the way I figure no amount of research or evidence would ever make some people give up their delicious bacon strips. The only way they will give up that toxic meat, is when they die an early death from eating the pig.

OUT OF THE BLUE

The blue oceans are not that blue anymore. They are becoming kind of gray because too many people use the oceans as a trash dump or even worse to dump raw sewage into it. The ocean has a cleaning mechanism in the currents, but the main cleaning mechanism of the ocean; is its army of bottom feeders. That army of bottom feeders includes the crabs, shrimp, lobsters, clams and all other shellfish. The more garbage there is the better fed and bigger the shellfish are.

Crabs and lobsters are bottom feeders; they eat the trash that goes to the bottom of the ocean. Clams, oysters, mussels and scallops are the filters of the ocean. These two groups are the janitors of the ocean. Shrimps are the cockroaches of the sea. They even look like cockroaches. Why would anyone want to eat sea cockroaches? I really do not know how some people will eat shrimp after shrimp without dropping down from a heart attack; not only are shrimp loaded with toxins they are also excessively high in cholesterol. I guess the body is stronger and more resilient than what I give it credit for.

Shell fish are so loaded with toxins; that scientists determine the toxicity of the sea by the level of toxins in shellfish. Plenty of people have died from eating shellfish, but even if people don't die from eating them they still ingest toxins in their bodies that will accumulate and eventually give them many health problems.

Pollution, dumped chemicals, fertilizers and just plain trash are destroying the plenty and nutritional value of sea food. I am beginning to be wary of eating anything from the ocean. Even fish that were completely healthy and nutritional are being ruined by the pollution in the seas. All the recent cases of dead fish floating and beached animals are symptom of the problems.

Another type of sea food that should not be eaten are predatory fish. The types of animals that full under the designation of predatory fish are Shark, Marlin, swordfish and some others. What is the problem with the predatory fish? The answer is simple, it lies in the concept of big fish eat little fish. You see in nature toxins and poisons travel up the food chain. When a bigger fish eats a smaller fish, the toxins and poisons of that little fish stay inside the big fish and the more little fish the predator eats the more toxins their body accumulates. Many of the predators are loaded with toxins and mercury in their bodies.

When a person eats a predatory fish, that person is eating the accumulated toxins, chemicals and what not from many other little fishes. Cooking well the fish will get rid of parasites, bacteria and maybe some viruses; but no amount of cooking will get rid of any toxins, poisons or chemicals. There is no way to clean these bad substances from a fish.

Well what animals are safe to eat from the ocean, well anything that has scales and fins is basically safe to eat. The scales and fins serve the fish to prevent the buildup of toxins in their bodies. If you think about it most of the sea life does have scales and fins so you can basically eat most of the ocean animals except for a few that have a task or role in removing poisons and toxins from the ocean environment that is the cleaning crew.

FRYING YOUR BRAIN

The cooking oils that we use to cook our foods are definitely bad for us. They appear to have a strong connection with heart disease and some cancers. All those cooking oils are also toxic and they add more fat to our already fat rich diet. The typical modern breakfast of fried eggs with fried ham and fried hash browns is plain crazy, eggs have their own fat, and ham is loaded with fat, why would anyone even think of adding more fat to them.

Don't believe the lies of the food industries that cooking oils are safe or good, they are not, those cooking oils are harmful to our health. All cooking oil contains about 120 calories per tablespoon. They are soaked in chemical solvents or heated to 122 to 200°F during the extraction process. They also contain bleaching agents, and are highly refined until they become transparent. The processing of oil strips it of most of its nutrients.

Some people fry everything in sight; they fry the beans, the rice, the meats and even the vegetables. Frying is perhaps the worst way to cook a meal, but the worst offense is to deep fry meats. Foods are never as viciously destroyed as in deep-frying. Foods can be cooked in many different manners. You can boil, steam, or roast your food.

The best advice is not to fry foods at all but if you must, then get oils which are unrefined and unfiltered. They still have all their nutrients, but most have a short shelf life, and of course they don't look as pretty as the oils sold in the stores. Yes it is more troublesome to get these oils but they are a whole lot better than what the supermarkets sell.

Olive oil and coconut oil seem to be the healthiest of the oils. These oils have a high smoke point, of over 410F degrees, and don't degrade as quickly as other oils do with repeated high heating. Studies have shown oxidation and hydrogenation occurs to a lesser degree in these oils than in others. Unfortunately these oils go rancid after a short time.

Deep-frying should be a crime; the oil products used for deep-frying are horrible. The high heat often used in deep-frying oxidizes the oil thereby producing free radicals, robs the food of nutrients and not to mention all the fires caused by the excessive heat.

Many people eat too many fried foods. They eat fried potatoes, fried rice and fried chicken. Come on chicken already has enough fat in itself, no need to add any more to it. They just keep on adding fat to the foods they eat, when they already have their own fat. If something is good then more of it should be better, right? Wrong, totally wrong.

When I go to eat I avoid any food that is fried. Instead of French fries, I get a baked potato or even better a small salad. If I get offered fried chicken I remove the outer layer, which is overloaded with fat. When offered something dripping with frying fat, I graciously turn it down or I just get a small portion.

What we need to do to have a healthy body and mind is to gather all those cooking oils and throw them into the garbage. That is exactly where they belong. Understand this, when you are frying your foods, you are also frying your brain.

MICROWAVE = MICRODEATH

The microwaving of food is perhaps the worst sin that can be committed against food. When you microwave food or reheat leftovers you are not only destroying the nutritional value of food, but you are also radically changing the molecular composition of the food you eat that is why microwave food tastes funny.

Before I get into the more technical details and the research that has been conducted on microwaved foods, I would like to appeal to the common sense and the wisdom of the body. The human body instinctively knows that it needs food, we are eating machines.

And for that the human body has senses, the sense of smell is one so is the sense of taste.

Seriously folks try this experiment on for size. Clean your teeth and your tongue; yes the tongue too, with a brush and then bite into a burrito or a piece of chicken that has been cooked in a regular oven. Just concentrate on how it tastes. Now do the same with a one that has been cooked in a microwave. Seriously do you think the human body wants microwaved food? If that is so why don't we get rid of all our stoves and just use the microwave to do all our cooking? If the microwave is not good for cooking food what makes anyone think it is OK to reheat food with it?

Not only that but all microwaves leak radiation that your body absorbs, the newer models produce less radiation than older models, but the problem remains that they still keep on producing harmful radiation and some of it leaks to the outside and if you are in front or around it you will get a small dosage. The microwave makers are aware of this issue but they dismiss it by saying the dosage is too small to cause any harm. Of course what they do not tell you is that the radiation accumulates in your body.

I do not have a microwave and I do not want to ever get one. I have studied the effects of long term radiation and I am fully aware of the risks involved. Why would I bring a death machine into my house? Of course I know it will not kill me instantly, it will just take some years of eating microwaved food before I start having all sorts of health problems. No thanks I pass on this convenience, I rather pop my popcorn the old fashion way.

The University of Minnesota strongly recommends not warming a baby's bottle in the microwave. It is obvious that a university must have knowledge of something wrong with that action otherwise why would a prestigious institution give that recommendation. The University has nothing to gain from giving that warning and might get sued by the makers of microwaves.

A scientist named Hans Hertel conducted some experiments of the effects of microwaved food in the human body. His conclusion was that such food causes a deterioration of the body. Every one of the participants in the experiment ended up with degenerative damage to their blood and their organs. Further research has indicated that the damage to the food is at the molecular level. So the food might look the same, but it is not the same it has been changed at the molecular level so the damage is invisible but the damage is there. Just because we do not see radio waves, germs or viruses does it mean they do not exist?

FROM BAD TO WORSE

In the desire to avoid the adverse health effects of bad substances people only go from bad to worse. Instead of abandoning the harmful substances or practices they seek to find substitutes. The solutions sometimes are worse than the initial problem.

Since some people have finally become convinced that sugar is a bad product; they have stopped eating regular drinks and begun drinking diet drinks. The problem is that those sugar substitutes are already beginning to bear their own claws, and the damage they do is not pretty. Let us just take a look at those substitutes.

Nutrasweet: This substance is horrible and harmful. It has been linked to cancer and other degenerative diseases. It only continues in the market due to the political power of the food industry.

Splenda: This is the newest star in the sweet world. It supposedly is a great substitute for sugar, but it already has been linked to serious health problems. I expect it will be withdrawn in a few years after it has killed its share of people.

Every single artificial sweetener has proven over time to be even worse than the sugar they replace. The effect from these artificial products does not show immediately but it is cumulative, so a few years pass before the effects show up.

Another area where substitutes are used is in cooking oils. They find out that some oils are bad and they go and use another kind of oil without realizing that the problem is not only the type of oils but it is also the method of getting those oils. As long as they fail to accept that the problem is also the processing of those oils, they will just keep on going on a merry go round going from one oil to another. Just look at some of the problems.

Lard. This is a pork product and it is harmful to the health. People used lard to fry for a long time, until finally people realized that it was not a good thing to do.

Vegetable oils. These were thought as great cooking oils but new research has shown that many people have health problems related to using those oils.

Hydrogenated fats: These were used for a while by the restaurants for deep frying, until now research has found there are many serious health problems with them.

Another product that was supposed to be bad for people was butter, but margarine turned out to be even worse. Recent studies show that butter is not harmful as long as it is made with organic milk and without any artificial ingredients. The problem was never butter, but the harmful substances added to it in the modern processing of butter.

Now let us go into the salt substitutes. Those salt substitutes are supposed to help people with high blood pressure to avoid salt, but this is another instance of the cure being far worse than the disease. All the salt substitutes are bad and none are good.

THE MODERN DIET

What is wrong with the modern diet? EVERYTHING. Just step into any market and see what people are buying for food, about 90 percent of what people buy is bad. The markets are only selling what people want, and that is junk food. That is because people are really ignorant of what good food is or they don't care. What is the result of eating a food that is 90 percent bad for us? How about a multitude of diseases.

Just walk into any food aisle in the supermarket and what do you see? Well the foods being sold have too much sugar, too much fat or too much salt. And if all that excess is not enough, just take a look at the fine print in the label description and you will see all kinds of unpronounceable chemicals and additives.

All those cereal boxes have so much sugar; they really belong in the candy aisle. Then they put the worst cereals at eye level to induce you to buy them. Then they have those pop tarts, pastries and the list goes on and on; the supermarket is a giant candy store.

They take those nutritious nuts and they shower them in salt, you can hardly find any peanuts or any other nuts without salt. They put enough salt in them to run a marathon. And let us not get started mentioning all the soups, crackers and other salty snacks.

What about the fat, there is enough extra fat in some foods to fry a couple of eggs. You grab some potato chips and your hands are dripping with all that grease and then some people dip those chips into fatty nacho cheese.

Of course let us not leave behind white flour. All those breads and pastries made with white flour have zero nutritional value. White bread is so devoid of nutrition that the government will not admit into its WIC nutritional program.

And let us not forget about all those nice chemicals. They even put those harmful chemicals in good food to preserve them. Those canned vegetables, which are marinated in all kinds of health destroying chemicals, are good for nothing but to fill the trash can.

Let us then take a look at the fast food restaurants and see that eating fast food will kill us really fast. Yes fast food = fast death. The typical lunch of hamburger, fries and coke, is so harmful, the only healthy thing to do is to throw it all into the trash.

We are surrounded with bad places to eat bad food. Donut shops, pizza places, and the list goes on and on. It is insane. Walk into any of those places and you will quickly see that you can hardly eat anything that will not hurt your health.

With our diet being so horrible no one needs to wonder why we as a society are so fat and why we are so plagued with so many diseases. We the enlightened modern society are very ignorant when it comes to our food. We are eating food that not even dumb animals will eat. We will eventually have to learn the hard way that a good diet does matter. We can't keep on eating this kind of diet and expect that everything will eventually turn our all right. This is not a nice truth or a happy truth, but it is the truth.

THE BIG PROBLEM

What is the big problem with obesity? Precisely that, being too big for our own good. It is estimated that over half of the people in America are overweight. This is definitively not good for our collective health.

What causes obesity? There are three main factors involved in obesity. The first is genes. Some people are genetically predisposed to gain weight. The second factor is diet. Eating a bad diet will surely get you fat, even if you come from skinny parents. The third factor is activity. If you do not burn those calories by regular activity or exercise, they will simply accumulate in your body.

Why do people eat so much food? Because we have an abundance of food and TV advertisers keep on pushing bad and unhealthful foods in front of our faces. The more food they sell the more money they make. Also some people turn to food as a source of comfort and happiness.

Why do people don't exercise? Because we have too many labor saving devices. We no longer have to walk anywhere. We also have mostly sedentary jobs, where we spend hours sitting on a chair. And to top it all off when we get home we tend to sit for hours on a comfortable couch.

What diseases are caused by obesity? There are many diseases caused or aggravated by obesity. The following is a short list.

Heart disease. The number one killer in America is caused or aggravated by excessive weight. There is also a strong link to hypertension another cause of heart problems.

Diabetes: Obesity obviously has a strong connection to this disease, 90 percent of diabetics are overweight

Arthritis: Excessive body weight worsens arthritis by putting stress on the joints, like the hips, knees and ankles.

Back problems: Excessive weight puts on a tremendous strain on the vertebral column with the lumbar region bearing the brunt of the weight.

Intestinal problems: The stomach and other internal organs were not meant to be overcrowded and overextended. Obese people have many gastrointestinal problems

Respiratory problems: Obese people are often short of breath. They sweat often on minor exertion or sometimes just suddenly.

Other problems: The list of problems related to obesity seems to get longer each year. It is now known that it is connected to some cancers and a host of mental problems.

With all these problems related to obesity, already well known why would people remain in that state is really beyond comprehension, it seems that good health is really not important to some people.

THE INVISIBLE KILLER

All electrical equipment causes electromagnetic radiation (EMFs). Everything from TV, radios, computers, cellular phones, microwave ovens, electric razors, electrical toys or whatever that is electrical, causes electromagnetic radiation. The body can handle radiation in small amounts, but it still remains to see if it can handle the massive amounts of radiation that comes from all our modern gadgetry.

Prolonged exposure to EMF is a big contributor to cancer, and it also debilitates the body. That is why people who work in front of a computer all day long are tired mentally and physically at the end of the day. Heavy users of the cellular phone suffer a higher incidence of brain cancer.

The idiot box is not only a colossal waste of time, but also a physical danger to our bodies. It is recommended that TV be viewed from at least ten feet away to avoid massive doses of radiation.

Computers can be great tools for work and achievement or they can also be another time drain in our lives, but they are definitely producers of magnetic radiation. Early computer monitors emitted too much radiation, but the new models are a little better. Of course you can also buy some special monitor screens that will absorb some of that excess radiation.

Of course the body is highly resistant and it can take some radiation, but what if you have all the lights on, then turn on the TV, or computer, then cook something in the microwave, and turn on the air condition to keep the heat down. Add to that a few phone calls and now we are talking a deathly dose of radiation going into your body.

You want to know how much radiation you are receiving just add up the amounts of radiation in your electronic gadgets and multiply it by the amount of time they are on and you will have a pretty good idea of how much radiation you are getting.

The problem is not only the amount of radiation but also the prolonged exposure to the radiation day after day. No wonder some people get tired in their own electrical wired homes. Their bodies are exhausted from fighting the electromagnetic effects. They need to go outdoors and get a breather.

The whole point is that the more electrical gadgets you have on the bigger doses of radiation you are receiving. Some of us probably are already past our limits. It is not wonder that some researchers are already finding links between the current wave of cancer diseases and our electrical gadgets. How long can your body receive these massive doses of radiation without developing cancer?

With more electronic gadgets coming our way I wonder what other effects will they have on our health and that of future generations. We might to wear radiation protective suits just to live in our own homes or we will we will have to increase our cancer donations a lot more. Welcome to the modern age of electromagnetic radiation, the invisible killer.

STRESS KILLS

Just what is stress? Stress is the body's response to an event. How you react to a threat or an unusual event is what causes stress. We need a certain amount of stress in our lives, but what we certainly do not need is an excessive amount of stress.

When you lose a job, have a sickness, someone moves away, or dies you are bound to develop some stress. However the amount of stress created in your body is different than that of another person. Everyone reacts to similar events in a different manner. To what a person is a major catastrophe to another it is a slight inconvenience. You are responsible for your level of stress; your reaction to an event is what determines the amount of stress you will have.

When a loved one dies, there is a lot of stress of dealing with all those feelings and the whole situation. It is not uncommon for people to have nervous breakdowns from all that stress. If you lose your job it is ok to feel bad about it, but after a couple of weeks that somber attitude has got to go. You have to go on and start looking for another job. It is perfectly ok to be human and react to bad events but there comes a point when you have get control back.

Stress causes physiological changes in your body. The body releases hormones like adrenaline and others in an attempt to deal with the situation that causes the stress. If your boss calls you and reprimands you, you will have an adrenaline release that should prepare you for your defense. If there is a fire or earthquake in the office you will also get an adrenaline response that should help you run for safety.

Stressful events will happen to everyone. But it is your response to those events that will determine how much affect they will have upon your physical health. You can not live in a state of constant alert, with your adrenaline and other hormones sky high. You have to learn how to deal effectively with stress, or the constant stress will hurt your body and eventually kill you. Yes there are effective ways to cope with stress.

The most important way to deal with stress is to remain in control and calm. The perfect medicine for stress is meditation and prayer. Believe it or not but prayer and meditation affect your physical health. The amazing thing about prayer and meditation is that they work regardless of which religion you practice. No wonder that prayer and meditations are a part of every religion.

Another way to deal with stress is by crying. Yes tears are great for stress relief, release tensions and they produce a cleansing effect from toxins that have accumulated in your body. Women and men need to weep in order to relieve internal emotional pain.

There are also some teas and herbs that can actually lower your stress level and calm you down. There are many types of stress relieving teas, the best way to find out which one works for you are through trial and experimentation. When some stressful event or bad thing happens, the best steps you can take is to remain calm, relax, pray, meditate, maybe cry a little and drink a nice hot tea.

NEGATIVITY

There is a problem that is not often addressed by the health advocates and that is negativity. Just what is negativity? It is anything that is negative, and that ranges from bad news to bad feelings and bad emotions.

You might not believe it but the news that you hear, see or read do affect your health. If you are constantly getting bombarded with tragic or bad news it will affect your mental and also your physical body. It will make you anxious, afraid and many other such similar reactions. That is why I tell people who are sick to stop getting the news. All that the news will do for you is to arouse your emotional state and make you sicker.

The biggest dosage of negativity often is internal. Some people tend to make themselves sick with all their constant brow beating of themselves. Internally they reproach themselves and say that they are not good. They are their own punching bag and whipping boy and lash out at themselves speaking and thinking all sorts of evil words, insults, and put downs.

Then there is life. All sorts of things happen to people, a dear family member dies, the company closes and lays everyone off. Someone lands in the hospital with a grievous disease. All those are negative feelings and emotions. You cannot go through life with constant worry, always angry at someone or with deep hatred for something.

All negative emotions anger, anxiety, depression, sadness, self-pity, shame, humiliation, regret, loneliness, guilt, frustration, and anything similar create poisons in your body that need to be kept in check. Because they will cause physical disease.

When somebody does your wrong and you carry a grudge, that grudge will eventually turn into hatred. All the accumulated hate will over time cause cancer or some other disease in your body. Get rid of your hatred before it gets rid of you. All you hatred will not do one bit of hurt to that person; it is you who will suffer from your own hatred.

The stories of people finding relief after forsaken negative emotions and feelings are many. When a sick person decides to forgive a past wrong, there is an internal relief and often a sudden recovery from some symptoms of the actual disease. There are countless stories of people getting healed from disease when they abandon their negativity.

Learn to relax, mediate and pray, learn to let go of negative emotions and negative feelings and your body will feel much better. I am sure you loved your family member much and miss that person, but your constant grief is not going to bring that person back, you have to continue living, remember the good times you had with that person not the fact that the person is gone.

It is estimated that over half of all diseases are the result of negative emotions or feelings. We need to find ways to unload all the negativity that surrounds us in the world. You might feel sorry for some people hurt in a natural disaster, but your feelings are not going to help them, they will need physical help, so write the check if you can help them. If your bank account is low, then simply realize that you cannot help them don't feel guilty for what you cannot do.

Your brain is part of your body, it is not a separate part and what you think does make a difference in your body below.

PART II: THE GOOD

THE BIG LIE

The big lie is that if you want to be healthy you will end up eating only lettuce and carrots. What a big fat lie! Don't you fall for that one. That is a lie propagated by fast food restaurants and all the other junk food merchants. They do it in order to discourage people from eating healthy and keep on eating their garbage and making them rich.

When you begin to eat healthy, you only are avoiding man processed foods. Like Jack Lane said, "if it is made by man don't eat it", he should know, after all when he died at the age of 96, he still was exercising and living an active lifestyle. You actually have more choices of natural food now that at any other time in history. You can get natural foods from all over the world.

There are many types of lettuces and also many types of carrots, but there are hundredths of vegetables besides lettuce and carrots. The supermarkets only carry the most popular items; they do not carry everything that is available. Yes there are over one thousand styles of salads; you could make a distinct salad for each day for over 3 years.

When it comes to fruits, there is a whole lot more than apples and the oranges. There are fruits that are popular in other countries, yet unknown in many others. You will be surprised at what you find in out of the way health food stores and ethnic markets. You will find fruits that you may never have seen before.

What about all those legumes and nuts. There are over two hundredth varieties of beans. And let us not forget about the grains. What you thought that all bread was just made with wheat? If you have not really tasted breads made with barley or other grains, you might be in for a pleasant surprise.

And let us not forget about the spices, there are hundredths of spices for making your food taste better. Or have you forgotten about that. Do you think sugar is the only sweetener there is? Come on wake up; don't let the sugar lobby cover your eyes to more healthful choices like honey, stevia or agave.

And what about the animals and fish? If you stop eating pork, do you think that cow and chicken are the only edible animals left to eat in the planet? Or that only salmon is fit to eat? Come on there are literally hundredths of species of land animals and fishes that you can eat, and what is great is that you can actually fish or hunt legally for some of them yourself.

Heck, there are things that people in other countries eat which are healthy, but some of us might be too squeamish to even consider. How about seaweed, yes people in Japan eat it. How about kangaroos, people in Australia eat them. How about buffalo meat? Yes you can get those and other meats if you know where to inquire.

Why the snide remarks, lies and mockery against those who want to eat healthy? Simple because the big corporations know that if enough people start eating healthy, their profits will begun to erode, so they try to make eating healthy as uncool as possible. That is why the big chains poke fun at people who care about their food, they know that the best way to destroy an idea is to make fun of it, to ridicule it and make it look silly.

THE PERFECT DIET

When people are warned of all the dangers in the modern diet they wonder what is there left to eat? Well the answer is everything. Yes EVERYTHING THAT IS NATURAL. You can eat vegetables, fruits, grains, legumes, nuts and meats yes even meats. The perfect diet is not one of deprivation but of abundance. To eat the perfect diet, just follow a few simple rules.

RULE ONE: The first rule of the perfect diet is, do not add anything. You have to eat what nature provides without adding anything to it. Do not add sugar, fat or salt. Natural foods have all the essential elements your body needs. And of course do not add any chemicals to your food. There is absolutely no need to add anything to your food.

RULE TWO: The second rule of the perfect diet is, eat a variety of foods. There is enough variety in nature to make millions of combinations of meals. Try mixing a little of this and a little of that. You will be delighted with some of the natural foods that you never have tasted before; there are plenty of little known natural foods.

RULE THREE: The last rule is, eat in small portions. Put small portions of your food in your plate or use a small plate and if you are still hungry snack on a fruit. We tend to eat more than what we actually need for our nutritional needs. The more you eat the bigger your stomach will physically grow and the more food it will need to get full.

SPICE IT UP: If eating natural foods seems too bland to you, you can add some natural spices. There is more to spices than just salt and pepper, there are hundredths of spices in the market. You can try different spices and see how you like them. You will be pleasantly surprised by the added taste some of these spices provide.

AVOID FAST FOOD: Avoid going to fast food restaurants, for mostly they sell foods that are bad. There is a very good reason why fast food is regarded as junk food. You will become discouraged because most of what they sell is bad. Avoid canned foods and TV dinners for exactly the same reason, they save you time but shorten your life.

GO FOR THE LEAST: When you go out to eat with some friends or they invite you to eat. Just remember to get the foods that have the least amount of sugar, fat or salt. If they offer you pizza, just get the smallest slice. If you are offered donuts get the plain one, without frosting or filling. Go for the least of the evils.

DON'T DIET: As a matter of fact don't waste your time and money reading all those diet books. No diet is a good diet. Forget about counting calories or carbohydrates. Forget about denial and deprivation. Forget about trying to remember which foods go together. All diets come and go they never last; people just jump from one harmful diet to another.

CHEAT A LITTLE: There is nothing wrong if you sneak in a small piece of chocolate, a cup of Java, a piece of cake, a fried leg, a ham sandwich or a small bag of pretzels once in a while. Your body can handle a little of those harmful substances as long as it doesn't become a daily habit. Total deprivation is not the goal of the perfect diet.

THE BIG CHALLENGE

Why do many people despair of eating and being healthy and just give up? Because society makes it really hard to be healthy. Everything is geared toward destroying our health. It is indeed a big challenge to buy healthy things for you life. You go to the supermarket and 90 percent of what you see is bad for you.

When you go to the market you see that everything either has too much sugar, too much fat or too much salt. Some people feel deprived because they can not buy everything that is available. The best option is to abandon the chain supermarkets and buy at the farmers market or the health food stores. There is no law that says you have to buy from the supermarkets, people who want to be healthy avoid the supermarkets.

Of course you might not want to abandon the supermarkets, in that case the trick is to be a smart shopper and go for the least of the evils. Read the labels and see which products contain the least amounts of sugar, fat, salt and other harmful additives, then write them down in a list, with their respective amounts. Once you have a list stick to buying only those products. Of course if healthier products come along then switch.

When you get to work and everybody hits the coffeepot, you go ahead and get some hot water and put in a bag of herbal tea. Instead of using sugar you use some honey to sweeten your tea. There is no reason why you can not take a tea break. You might have to bring in healthy snacks like fruits or nuts to avoid hitting the snack machine.

Of course bringing in healthy food from home, might not be the standard practice at your workplace, but think of all the money you will save by avoiding the fast food joints. Of course if there is a festivity or people are going out to eat lunch as a team then go ahead and buy a salad or the least harmful of the meals in the menu. Plenty of restaurants have a nutritional guide; even McDonalds has a nutritional chart, so use it.

Advertisers want you hooked on TV, so you watch more commercials so they can sell you more junk food. Their programs are not made for your benefit but for their benefit. Get the TV guide and highlight only those programs you want to watch and stick with it, don't fall for the teasers.

Get of the couch and go to the gym. Go out there into the world and have a healthier lifestyle. Take up a sport or do something that improves your health. Maybe take a cooking class so you can stop buying all those harmful foods. If you are going to play video games, set a timer in top of the video game console and check it once in a while. Set time limits or amounts on whatever passive fun you are having.

Living a healthier lifestyle might mean going against the current and standing out a little. You might be the only person drinking water while others are drinking that sugary poison. You will be out there in the gym while others are home watching some idiotic sitcom or reality program. It might be a little strange to be the odd person, but it's worth it, for it will help you to achieve success in your career and life.

THE NATURAL WAY

When people find out how deadly the food in the supermarket really is, they wonder, if there is anything they can eat. Yes there is you can go ORGANIC. No, this is not some New Age jumbo numbo, it is the way the people in biblical times used to eat and people have eaten for centuries throughout the world; and many people still do.

ORGANIC MEANS NATURAL. Organic means foods grown without genetic manipulation, artificial fertilizers or deadly pesticides. You just have to accept the fact that organic fruits and vegetables will not look perfect with no scratches or any blemishes for that is not naturally possible, but they are healthy. Of course since organic foods are labor intensive, naturally they are bound to cost a little more.

Organic produce is a whole lot healthier than the supermarket produce. They have many strong factors in their side. They are loaded with vitamins and minerals. They have no genetic manipulation, they have no artificial fertilizers and they have no deathly pesticides. You can eat them without fear and will be much healthier. If you are sick just the fact of switching to an organic diet will help you to heal faster and better.

This also including switching to organic meats and dairy products. The modern animal rearing practices are also totally unnatural. Cows and other animals are fed growth hormones and antibiotics in order to fatten them. Chickens cooped up in tiny cages, being overfed hormones and tricked into laying more eggs, no wonder we are sick.

Another point is that foods grown by big farmers tend to be heavily subsidized by the government, while organic farms get little support from the government. The reason is quite simple, big farmers can grow a whole lot more of their nutrition deficient products at a lower cost.

Now let us think about this, we have an abundance of food, yet we are undernourished. We should be the healthiest people since we have so much food, but unfortunately that is not how it works out. We are plagued with all kinds of nutritional diseases. We have given up the natural way and taken the artificial way and now we are paying for it with our health. We keep on eating all the artificially grown and produced foods, and then we want to take artificial vitamins to make up the deficiencies, how idiotic.

We get sick from the foods we eat, shouldn't that cause a bell to ring in the head. "Hey perhaps we are doing something wrong, but no, that is not what we do, we want the doctor to shoot up us with some magical drugs to take away the pain and the multi-billion dollar drug companies are only happy to oblige.

You may complain and say that you cannot afford organic foods, but think of it this way. You will have to eat more artificially grown foods to get the same nutrients in organic goods, you will have to buy expensive vitamins to complement your diet, and you will visit the doctor more often (Medicine is expensive). Of course let us not forget about the effects of those deadly poisons and chemicals. Now tally it all up and see which food is really expensive.

NUTRITION

Now why is nutrition important? Because whatever you eat gets broken down by the body and is absorbed into your body; yes you are what you eat. If your body is properly fed then your body and your mind will function at optimum levels. When your body feels great then your mind will also feel great. Good nutrition allows you to have a healthier body and mind and live life more fully.

IT AFFECTS THE BODY: Nutrition is important to a well functioning body. Improper nutrition will cause fatigue and in your body. You will feel sluggish and your work pace will slow down to a crawl, and you will accomplish little.

IT AFFECTS THE MIND: Bad nutrition is at the root of mental fatigue and confusion. If your mind lacks the proper amount of vitamins and minerals, it will not be able to focus on important matters and you will make many mistakes and accidents.

IT CAUSES DISEASE: There are many diseases that are caused or aggravated by poor nutritional choices. Scurvy is one disease that can be cured by eating citrus foods like lemons, oranges and grapefruits.

IT WILL GET YOU FAT: If the foods you eat are loaded with fats and sugar your body will just incorporate them into the body as fat. The body is designed to store energy. It is a natural mechanism that protects it against starvation and emergencies.

BAD AND EXCESSIVE: Not only do people eat too many of the wrong foods, they eat an abundance of them. They ask for the double burger and then super-size the fries and the coke. They double scoop the ice cream and get a giant bar of candy.

THE DIET BUST: Some people decide to lose the fat and go on fad diets. The problem is that fad diets only make the problem even worse. Diets work on the principle of deprivation and drastic changes and no one likes deprivation or drastic food changes.

THE RIGHT WAY: The only way to adopt proper nutrition is to make gradual changes into your diet. Substitute one bad food for a good one, then wait about three weeks or until you are used to the change before introducing another change.

TAKE SUPPLEMENTS: If you eat a proper diet, you probably don't need any supplements. Unfortunately most people do not eat a proper diet and they need to augment their nutrition with solid or liquid vitamin and minerals supplements.

GET PROFESSIONAL HELP: If you have trouble or need help with your nutrition then see a certified nutritionist. Just be careful for there are some wild fanatics advocating all kinds of crazy ideas. Some of their weird advice will hurt your health or even kill you.

EAT YOUR WAY TO SUCCESS: If you eat the proper foods your body will be full of energy that lasts throughout the day. You will have less health problems and you will have more time to dedicate to doing your job right and living life fully.

COMMON SENSE IN NUTRITION

Eating right does not take a PhD, or spending years becoming a nutritionist. It only takes some common sense. Listen to nature and your body; they know what is best for you. We humans think we can improve on nature, but we only end up destroying the foods that are good for us and damaging our bodies.

EAT NATURAL FOODS: Nature has already provided plenty of the foods you need to stay healthy. Yes this means eating plenty of raw vegetables, fruits, grains and nuts. Raw foods plucked out of the tree or plants are the best. Any illiterate native knows that nature provides for our nutrition foods that are good.

COOK THEM RIGHT: Obviously some natural foods can not be eaten raw. Foods like the potato, beans, wheat, spinach, cabbage and others. They would harm us if we don't cook them, and take away some of their hardness, acids and other harmful substances, but when foods are overcooked or cooked wrong some of the nutrients are lost in the process.

AVOID OVER-PROCESSED FOODS: Some foods like bread, tortillas, cheese, yogurt and others are obviously processed by men. Nature does not produce them on its own; we have to make them. But the more refinement is done to the food the more it loses some of its nutrients. That is one reason why white flour is bad, it has been over-processed.

CHEMICALS ARE NOT FOOD: All the preservatives and additives put into packaged foods were never meant to be eaten. They do not exist in natural foods; they were created in laboratories and then added to foods. Most of them are carcinogens and poisons to our bodies. These chemicals are the probable cause of many modern diseases.

EAT ONLY WHEN YOU ARE HUNGRY: Your body is the best indicator of when you should eat. Let your body set the timetable as to when and how often you should eat. Don't go by tradition or social norms. Maybe you need to eat only two meals or perhaps you need to eat four times per day, let your body decide.

EAT UNTIL YOU ARE FULL: Once again let your body decide when it is full, and stop that nonsense of counting your food. No, you do not have to finish all the food in your plate if you are full. If you are still hungry then get a little more. Your stomach knows when it has had enough and will send a signal to the brain to stop when it is time to stop.

ENJOY YOUR MEAL: Go ahead, relax and enjoy your meal. Take the time to taste and chew the food. If you don't like a certain food just put it aside and leave it. Eating should be a pleasurable experience not an endurance test. If you are angry, upset or nervous calm down before you eat, those strong emotions will interfere with the digestion.

EAT THE SWEETNESS OF NATURE: If you got a sweet tooth, don't worry nature has provide treats for you; fruits, nuts and honey. Fruits have fructose, this is the good sugar that nature intended for us to eat, but you need to eat the whole fruit. When fruits are juiced the skin and the fiber is discarded and their valuable nutrients are lost. The fiber in the fruit is there for a reason.

FRESH IS BEST

Fruits and vegetables need to be eaten fresh in order to get their full nutritional value, and avoid sickness. This means getting these foods in their seasons. There is a proper time when fruits and vegetables are at their best. If you buy too early in the season you will get tasteless foods, and if you buy too late in the season you will get overripe foods.

This same advice applies to meats. The fresher the meat the better it will be for your health. If the meat smells or doesn't look right forget about buying it, it probably has begun to rot. Frozen meats just can't compete with fresh meats. You just can't beat the taste of fish recently caught.

If you can raise some of your own foods then do it; it just takes a little time and effort. There are some farmers who will allow you to pick your own fruits and vegetables. There are also places where you can choose the live animals you want and they will butcher them for you. If you live close to nature you can go hunting or forage for wild foods (of course you must really know what you are getting or risk poisoning yourself). And if you live by the ocean or a river then you can go fishing. Talk about fresh food!

Canning is done to preserve the excess of the harvest, but the whole canning process destroys vitamins and nutrients in the food. Vegetables are soaked in preservatives and fruits are drowned in sugary syrups. The only place to put canned foods is in big can, better known as the trash can.

Freezing foods might be better than canning but they still loose nutrients. It is best to buy frozen foods last and put them away first, so they will not thaw and allow bacteria to multiply. Frozen foods also lose much of their flavor and texture.

Drying and pickling are much better than canning or freezing. These two processes have been used for centuries to keep food for the long winter months and so far they have an excellent record. Sun drying is the best method of drying foods and vinegar is the best for pickling. Keep your dried foods away from moisture and pests.

You need to keep your foods in their proper place to keep them fresh. That is why refrigerators come with special compartments for vegetables and fruits so that they will keep longer without spoiling. Don't leave eggs, milk or other perishables too long out of the refrigerator. The longer they are out the more chances that they will grow bacteria.

You need to eat the oldest foods or throw them away. Never eat foods past their expiration date, yes they could still be good but why take the chance on getting food poisoning. Yes I have eaten sometimes things that have expired but only if it is one day or two, I do not want to take chances with my health. It is cheaper and easier to buy new foods than to go to the hospital or the cemetery.

The longer food sits in the shelf or the refrigerator the more chances that it will expire, get moldy or spoil. As food ages it begins to lose flavor and nutrients. One trick is to write in labels the date the foods are bought and then put the labels on the foods. Use big letters in the labels so that the expiration date can be seen even if the item is in the back of the fridge. Another trick is to use color labels. There are many other tricks people can use to keep foods fresh longer.

WHOLE FOODS, WHOLE BODIES

The ancients ate whole foods and had whole bodies, however we have gotten away from that and now we have partial foods. We no longer eat whole grains like whole wheat, or whole rice, neither do we eat whole foods, and sure enough we suffer from all kinds of nutritional deficiencies and diseases.

Instead of eating whole wheat, which is healthful, we now eat white flour, which is totally devoid of nutrients; full of empty calories and it also contains traces of bleaching agents. The nutritionally deficient white flour is used in bread, pizza, donuts, tortillas, and many other products. Just a look at the back of the package if it just says flour, you can bet it is white flour. If it does not say "whole wheat" it is simply not good.

Instead of eating whole rice, which is healthful, now we eat that polished white rice which is also almost totally devoid of nutrients. People eat bowls full of rice that only make them fat and gives them the beriberi disease. Then to get well they buy expensive vitamins, when the easiest solution would be to eat the whole rice.

Instead of eating whole fruits, we now squeeze them into sugary drinks. Fruits were made to be eaten whole with the fiber, the fiber in the fruits are not there just to take up space, they are there because they aid in the digestive process. Juicing of fruits or vegetables is unnatural and a waste of vital nutrients, fiber and other vital substances that our bodies need.

We keep on refining and taking away from foods their completeness. All these modern refinements leave foods nutritionally deficient. All these refined foods are making us fat and sickening our bodies. We are destroying that which is good in some misguided attempt to get purer foods, without comprehending that we need the whole food.

A devious trick is the so-called "enriched or fortified" foods, but if you look past this trick you will see that the foods are still deficient. Enriched or fortified sounds like a healthy thing, but it only means that they put back some of the original vitamins. What the manufacturers forget to mention is all the other components that were subtracted from the original foods and not put back in. These foods are still incomplete foods.

The reason that people prefer white bread, white rice, concentrated juices and other refined foods is because those products taste better. That is all; so we prefer to eat something that tastes good instead of something that is nutritious. We are like children who want to eat candy instead of what is good for our bodies. What a sad state of affairs!

"Come on white flour, white rice or other refined foods are not as bad as sugar or fat." Just because these foods are not as bad as refined sugar, fat or other harmful substances, does not make them harmless. They might take longer to hurt your system, but they will definitely hurt it. It is like asking which poison would you prefer one that kills you in weeks, one that takes a few months or one that takes a few years, they all will kill you.

What are we to do? Simple we need to go back to eating whole foods. We need to go back to eating whole grains, whole wheat, whole rice, whole fruits and whole vegetables.

THE RAW DEAL

What is the best way to eat fruits, vegetables and nuts? The best way is to eat them raw. When you eat raw foods you are getting the maximum nutrition possible. And not only do you get great nutrition, but you also get strong healthy fiber into your system. Of course you can not eat raw meats, legumes or grains; they do need to be cooked. And it is perfectly ok to cook them.

Any heat applied to the vegetables will destroy some of the vitamins. The most healthful way to cook vegetables is to steam them, but even with this process the vegetables still lose some nutrients. That is why it is always better to eat them raw. If you boil vegetables do not throw away the vitamin rich water, but use it to cook the rice or some other dish.

Not only do vegetables lose nutrients with cooking, but also the fiber that is so good for our bodies becomes less useful. The fiber from the vegetables will help your digestive system process the food better. That is why a salad is always more healthy than a plate of steam vegetables.

Fruits should never be cooked. When fruits are cooked, the glucose in the fruit becomes highly concentrated and the fiber is totally destroyed. Some people cook fruits without realizing the harm they are doing to their nutritional value.

Peanuts and a few other nuts can be eaten raw, but some are toasted to take away the bitter flavor and that is perfectly OK, but that should be the extent of the cooking. To eat walnuts, pecans and other nuts all you have to do is crack them open. Nuts have high concentrations of vitamins and good fats, and are perfect for snacks and salads.

You might not be used to eating much raw foods, but it is only a matter of getting used to it. People for centuries have eaten raw foods. There are plenty of cultures where people still eat plenty of raw foods and few items are cooked.

It would be great for your health if you ate only raw vegetables, fruits and nuts, but it is not necessary to maintain good health. If you can eat at least one raw meal per day then you should be in great health. How about eating a salad for lunch or dinner? Or perhaps a bowl of fruit for breakfast? Perhaps add some raw nuts to your morning cereal? You could also add some raw foods along with your cooked meal; OK at least eat raw foods as snacks.

No I am not advocating that you should only eat raw foods, I am not a hard core raw food faddist, but I insist that you do need some raw foods in your daily diet, you can not keep on eating only hot meals for every meal and expect your digestive system to work right, it is not going to happen.

And it is not only the heat that hurts the nutrients in vegetables and fruits, but also the cold. If you don't believe it, just try freezing a banana and then eating it. The freezing process will destroy some of the nutrients. So it appears that these foods do not like it when it is too hot or too cold. If you like exotic raw foods, with our modern transportation systems getting raw foods from far away regions should not be a problem.

MULTIPLYING YOUR NUTRITION

I think the perfect way to have excellent nutrition is by multiplying your nutrition. How can you multiply your nutrition? Well simply by embracing the principles of complementing, diversity and mixing. These principles take some time to understand and put into practice but well worthy to learn them.

The first principle is to complement your meal. Per example, you can eat for breakfast one egg, some beans and bread or tortillas with a glass of milk for a juice drink. This breakfast is great for you have proteins, fiber, grains, and dairy foods in one meal. You just have to learn the proper combinations of foods that will give you the best nutrition possible. To have better nutrition you need to learn which foods complement each other to create a total meal, you need meals that are balanced.

Another great principle is diversifying your meals. This means try to eat different meals every day. Have a different breakfast every day, a different lunch and a different dinner. By having a variety of foods through the week you increase the nutritional value of your meals. This way your body will never develop any vitamin or mineral deficiency.

Another principle is to mix your meals. The principle of mixing is not that complicated. It is simple the mixing of foods types of the same kind. Instead of having just regular bread, how about eating multi-grain bread. You could try eating 12-grain bread. How about eating bean soup with different types of beans, after all there are over 200 varieties of beans.

There are many ways to mix food items. Instead of eating plain oatmeal try 10-grain oatmeal. Instead of eating simple lettuce in your salad try putting more than one type of lettuce in your salad. You can try making a fish soup made of more than one kind of fish. Or you could make soup of chicken, turkey and duck.

Think of how beautiful, colorful and nutritional a bowl of vegetables or fruits are. Try to get as many different combinations as you can. One day you can make a tropical fruit salad, while at another time you could try to make a vegetable soup just of purple or yellow vegetables. Learning how to multiply your nutrition takes some time, but it is fun to experiment with different combinations.

Do you know that in different countries people eat different breakfasts, lunch and dinners. Have you ever had a French day, where all your meals are typically dishes from France? Perhaps you can try a Japanese or Cajun day and eat like the Japanese or Cajuns eat everyday. The whole point of this is to broaden you gastronomical world and understand that there are a whole lot of different foods and food combinations that perhaps you haven't even thought of.

These ideas of complementing, diversity and mixing are not only great to experience and experiment with but their diversity can provide many health benefits. Your body will get a rich mix of vitamins, minerals and other nutrients. And the best benefit of it is that you will break free from the idea that you can not eat healthy and have fun and also lay to rest the myth that to eat healthy you have to confine yourself to eating carrots and lettuce.

THE BIG DIFFERENCE

Two items could be called by the same name and even look alike but there could be a big qualitative difference between them. There is a difference between Idaho potatoes and potatoes raised elsewhere. There is a difference between Florida oranges and oranges raised elsewhere. People who do not understand this concept think that sugar is sugar, fat is fat, and salt is salt. They don't understand the differences.

All foods are not the same. Sugar and honey both are sweeteners but it is clear that honey is superior to sugar. Vegetables and animals both have fat, but it is clear that vegetable fat is better than animal fat. Salt from marshes is vastly superior to salt from mines. Brown rice is much better than white rice. Organic apples are better than regular apples. Fertile eggs are better than non-fertile eggs. Cheeses from one place are better than cheeses from another place. And the examples could go on and on.

You need to understand that the differences are also created by how things are created even when dealing with the same product. Chicken meat varies in quality according to what the chicken was fed, how it was raised and whether it was given hormones. There is a big nutritional difference but most people just buy chicken under the impression that one piece of chicken is the same as another piece, without realizing that one chicken could be healthy and nutritious while the other is less healthy and nutritious.

Once you understand and accept this concept of qualitative differences in foods of the same kind, you will be on your way to better health. You will start buying foods on which ones are better rather on which ones are cheaper or which ones are more promoted.

Don't be the clueless person who thinks that all wheat bread is the same, they are all different.

What you have to consider is where the products come from. There are some areas more suited than others for growing or raising some products. Another thing is what was the animal or plant fed. Was the plant given natural fertilizers or artificial ones? Was the cow fed with good fresh grass, dry grass or grain? How the plants and animals were raised; were the plants showered with pesticides or were the animals raised in cages. In short everything that was done to the plants or animals has a direct effect on the quality of the food product.

Perhaps this will help you to avoid some traps that unscrupulous food makers do. Some will sell brown sugar, which really is white sugar with coloring added. Some will sell brown rice, which in reality is regular white rice with coloring added; and the tricks by these dishonest merchants just go on and on. You are not buying what you think you are buying because they play games with words and labels. Some will claim low in fat or low in sugar, but if you look carefully in the labels you will see worse substitutes.

Don't buy food items in low nutritional value. You need to be selective so that you can buy that which is healthy and good. Yes it takes a little time to know the difference between a good hamburger and a bad one, but it is time well spent. You be informed, you be different, you be smart, know the big difference and your body will thank you for it.

ANIMALS MEATS

I want to dispel the myth that animal meat is bad to eat, it is not. Of course this goes totally against the beliefs of vegetarians even the hard core "vegans". With my sincere apologies to them I will state the following; there is nothing wrong with eating animal meat, as long as it is eaten in small portions and you follow certain rules.

For those of you who want to try out the vegetarian lifestyle, you have my best wishes for your health. You will probably be a little healthier for it. However be aware that people who become vegetarians run the risk of having nutritional deficiencies, and also be low on vitamin B12; usually it is because they are not informed of those risks.

For the rest of you who like me do not want to give up meat, I will state that there is no need to feel guilty or feel that we can not be healthy because we are meat eaters. Of course this does not mean that you should just eat any type of animal or in any amount. There are certain animals you should not eat and also you need to eat meat in moderation.

The animals that we should never it are those which are classified as dead matter eaters. That includes all the scavengers and predators. That list includes the pig, the vulture, the eagle, shrimp, shellfish and similar ones. In other words anything that survives by eating garbage or by killing and eating other animals. In other words we will stick with eating only animals that eat vegetation and for sea animals anything that has scales and fins.

Meat is good; it is full of proteins and other good nutrients. You can eat most meats with no problem. You can eat chicken, beef, lamb, goat and deer. You can eat the meat of any animal that has been accepted as proper for human consumption, as long as the meat is not spoiled and comes from a clean slaughterhouse.

There are some farmers who still raise their animals in an organic manner without loading them up with growth hormones or shooting them full of antibiotics. If you can find organic meat then by all means buy it, for it is the best. Or at least buy fresh meat, there are some places where they will slaughter the animal that you choose.

There are just a few of rules about eating meat.
1. If you can afford to get kosher meats then get it
2. Do not eat the blood of animals for it is full of toxins, wash the meat good.

3. Get lean cuts only or get a knife and cut out the excess fat of animals
4. Eat it in small portions, too much meat creates an excess of uric acid.
5. Meat has some natural fat, so don't fry your meats; they will absorb more fat.

Why I recommend kosher meat, simple because it is meat where the animal has been slowly bled to death. Blood is a cleansing agent; it carries and accumulates toxic substances. As the blood travels thorough the body it gathers all the toxins that the animal body has rejected. The circulatory system acts like a sewer system and bleeding empties those poisons from the meat. For meat to be considered kosher it has to be certified by a competent authority.

In the old times people used to raise their own animals, and animals that were butchered were sold immediately, but that is not longer possible for most people. Now days you have to make sure that you buy fresh meat. The longer the meat has been on display the worse the meat is. Refrigeration can delay the spoiling process, but eventually the meat will spoil. Freezing will not keep meats forever either.

Another way to get meat is to go hunting, just like in the old times. You can go into the wilderness and hunt many animals. Of course you might need a hunting permit and abide by the rules. There are plenty of wild game and birds still available.

A good thing to keep in mind is that in ancient times most people only ate meat on special occasions or only a little of it. People would go hunting and then dry meat and eat it in small portions through the months Eating an abundance of meat was not an everyday occurrence like in modern times. One final thought, I am not opposed to eating meat at all, but seriously folks today we eat too much darn meat protein.

DAIRY PRODUCTS

There is no problem in eating animal products like eggs, milk or cheese. But there are some issues and rules that need to be followed with dairy products. The first and most important rule is that dairy products should be **organic**. That is supremely important.

Now let me state clearly and emphatically that no baby should be given cow's milk. Their stomachs can not handle the protein in the milk. The only milk that is healthy for a baby is the mother's milk. After the child is one or two years old then cow or goat milk can be introduced into the diet until adolescence.

MILK: Milk is good for children, not for adults. I do not care what the dairy companies say or what scary commercials they show on TV, grown adults seldom should drink milk and only in small amounts. Have you ever seen any other mammal in nature drink milk after it has grown up? Store milk is the worst type of milk; it has been homogenized and made unfit to drink. The best milk is raw organic milk, if it is not raw or organic, throw it out.

CHEESES: Some cheeses are better than others are because of what milk was used to make them. There is a big difference between cow's milk and goat's milk. There is also a big difference in what kind of cows the milk comes from. Another important factor is how is the cheese prepared. Some are smoked, others have too much salt added, and others have too much fat. You need to how know the cheese is prepared and what ingredients were used in it before you put it in your body.

CREAMS: Sour creams come in different varieties; the same issues that apply to cheese also apply to creams. Read the labels to know exactly what is in the product and ask questions before you start putting in down your throat.

YOGURTS: Yogurt is excellent as long as it is not loaded with sugar. I can assure you that you will not find any healthy yogurts in the local store. They are all bad for you. The only place you can find any good yogurt is the one that you make yourself or in some health food stores.

EGGS: Eggs are full of protein and unfortunately cholesterol. There is a good reason for that. The yolk contains a lot of cholesterol because it is meant to provide nutrition to the growing chick for many days. When you eat the egg, you are eating what an embryo chick would eat over several days. That is why you need to limit your consumption of eggs and also don't fry your eggs, they are already loaded with their own fat. Of course your eggs should be organic fertile eggs. Why? Because they are the best for your health. You won't find healthy eggs in the supermarket; you have to go to a health food store.

There is nothing wrong with drinking raw organic milk; that is the only kind I seldom drink; but to tell you the truth, you really do not need to. Despite all the propaganda about calcium deficiency, you really do not need to drink milk. Have you ever seen mammals in the wild suffering from osteoporosis or calcium deficiency? Once they are grown they do not drink any milk. The only thing they drink is water and the only things they eat are natural herbs.

DRINK AND BE MERRY

You were made to drink water, your body functions best with water. Water cleanses your system and keeps you healthy, and yes that is a fact. You were not made to drink other substances. You were definitely not made to drink sodas, sugary fruit juices or other unhealthful drinks. The kidneys filter any impurities in the water, they are great filters, but they were not created to filter out the massive amounts of sugar and chemicals in modern drinks. No wonder many people suffer from kidney diseases.

The worst drink in the whole wide world without a doubt has to be the cola drinks. They are overloaded with refined sugar. Have all kinds of cancer causing chemicals, and also contain acids that eat the lining of the stomach and cause havoc with stomach acids. And let us not forget about the high concentration of caffeine in many of them.

Nothing beats water as a hydrator. Not the sugary drinks or even those sport drinks. Those sport drinks hydrate the body at a price. They pump up the system with an overdose of salt and harmful substances. Athletes are able to absorb the harm from those substances because they are at peak physical shape. Their bodies are strong and efficient machines and can handle it. But most people do not have an athlete's body.

Many people taste water and find it bland and tasteless, that is exactly how it is suppose to taste. Water is supposed to be colorless, odorless and tasteless. They are so used to colorful sugary liquids that water just is not exciting. Water is not supposed to be exciting it is supposed to support your life. Of course you can add a slice of lemon to flavor it.

What about alcohol? Your body was definitely not made to drink alcohol. Yes the body can handle a small amount of alcohol with no problem, but your body can not handle the massive amounts of alcohol in most beers and wines. The liver synthesis the alcohol and filters it. That is why cirrhosis of the liver is quite common among alcoholics.

Having said all that I am not one that advocates total abstinence. There have been times when I have been invited to a celebration or two. In those times, I graciously take a small cup of wine and take a sip or two. It really is in bad manners and taste to scold the hosts for serving alcoholic beverages. If you believe in total abstinence, well good for you, when the wine is being served just turn your glass upside down. Please do behave like a civilized person not like an idiot; a party is not the time or the place to give a lecture on the evils of drinking.

The ancients often drank water mixed with wine because their water was often not pure. The alcohol in the wine killed any dangerous germs. Of course that is not longer a problem with our modern means of filtration. Germs are totally wiped out and water is made drinkable. The problem is that now we are going in the opposite direction. When water is totally distilled, important minerals are removed from the water. That is why it is dangerous to drink distilled water, because it is free of needed minerals.

Another thing to avoid is regular tap water, the water has been chlorinated to kill the germs, but the chlorine has not been removed. The water is free of germs but full of chlorine; I often wonder which one is worse. Only drink water that has been purified, get a good filter and put a label on it with the date when the filter needs to be changed.

For a nice treat or change of pace try drinking mineralized water. Also once in a while you can drink a water diluted pure fruit juice, but make sure that no sugar is added to your fruit juice. Although I totally advice against it, if you really feel you must have a soda, then make it one without caffeine, fill up your cup to the top with ice and don't refill it.

MORE DRINKS

Although water is the best drink for your health you do not have to confine yourself to drinking just water in its many variations. There are plenty of drinks you can make yourself that are healthy and do not harm your body.

What about juicing? Fruits were made to be eaten whole. Juicing destroys the fiber in fruits and produces a highly concentrated and unhealthy amount of fructose. The stomach has a hard time absorbing such a high concentration of fructose. And to make matters worse some people add sugar to their juices.

However that does not mean that you can not indulge once in a while. Just remember that some fruit juices are too sweet and need to be diluted in some water otherwise you get a full blast of fructose. Your body has no problems handling small amounts of these juices, but you can not make this an every day meal experience.

Some people like to drink vegetable juice, which I consider an excellent source of vitamins and minerals. You can try many combinations of vegetable juices. However just like with fructose the body does not like high concentration of these kinds of substances so it is best to drink them in small amounts or diluted with some water.

There are hundredths of fruits to make juices from; there is no need whatsoever to buy sodas, or any of the sugary drinks in the market. There is no reason except for the lack of knowledge that people are drinking all those awful harmful drinks in the market.

Orange juice, grapefruit and lemonade are very popular and yes they are healthy, but not on an empty stomach. The orange and grapefruit juices should be without any added sugar or additives. The lemonade can be sweetened with xylotol, fructose, stevia or other natural sweeteners. These citric fruits have strong acids so go easy on them.

Coconut water is another excellent drink. It is all natural and very healthy. You just have to get the coconut when they are in their season, otherwise if they are overripe their flavor is a little tart and their nutritional value begins to decline.

Teas are excellent for drinking and there are a great variety of them. Black teas have a high concentration of caffeine but not as much as coffee. Green teas are low in caffeine and they have excellent anti-oxidants. However there are a whole lot of herbal teas that contain no caffeine and have many refreshing and healthful qualities.

You can also drink dairy products; some of the best are raw milk, goat milk, and also kefir. In some places you can get camel's milk or the milk from other animals. If your stomach can not handle raw milk then boil the milk, let it cool and then drink it.

There are many other drinks made from different foods or cereals. Some drinks are rice based, others use corn and others use some other grains or natural ingredients. Some are drunk hot and others cold, some are well known while others are not. Any drink that you make is bound to be much healthier than whatever sells in the supermarket.

NATURAL SWEETENERS

Refined sugar is a harmful and bad sweetener, however most people think that it is the only sweetener or that the only alternatives are the artificial sweeteners that cause cancer and other horrible diseases. Well they are totally misinformed and do not know of the many healthful alternatives. Of course the sugar industry would like to keep people in this ignorance and the artificial sweeteners companies have a nice niche market.

Honey is excellent as a replacement for sugar. It has been used for centuries and is widely available. The darker the honey the better tasting it is. Bees produce different flavors of honey depending on which flowers they use. Honey has nutrients and trace minerals. It also has a lower glycemic index than sugar. Pound by pound honey is much sweeter than sugar so you have to use less.

There are some products that come from the same source as refined sugar, but they are not as harmful. These are brown sugar, blackstrap molasses, rapadura, sucanat, turbinado sugar and evaporated cane sugar. Of course some dishonest merchants add coloring to regular sugar and then sell it as brown sugar, so unless you know the source, avoid brown sugar. All the others are basically cane sugar that have not been as heavily processed and stripped of its nutrients or refined to the extent that refined sugar has been.

Of course not all the sweeteners come from the sugar cane or beets; there are other sources of sweeteners. A little known but excellent sugar replacement is stevia. This comes from a plant in South America and it is a lot healthier than sugar. The sugar industry has fought the introduction of stevia and has attempted to squash any publicity about it. The sugar industry considers it a threat to their empire.

Agave comes from a cactus plant and is another little known sweetener that is excellent as a replacement for sugar. It is rich tasting and full of vitamins and minerals. The glycemic index is very low and it causes no harmful effects on the body. I consider it an excellent substitute for refined sugar.

Another substitute is xylitol; this is a sugar derived from fruits and vegetables. It has many advantages, like it doesn't leave an after taste, it is lower in calories and it is safe for diabetics. The only problem is that in large amounts it has been known to produce such symptoms as bloating, flatulence, and diarrhea.

We can continue the list with brown rice syrup, Maple syrup, and some others less known. The point I am trying to make is that basically anything else is better than refined sugar or those cancer producing synthetic sugars. The sugar industry would like to make people believe that there are not good alternatives to their product or that a sugar is a sugar and it doesn't matter where it comes from.

Anyone who says a sugar is a sugar is ill informed, ignorant or doesn't really understand how the body process sugar. Let me explain you to that it does matters how much sugar you put into the body, but it also matters how fast or slow the body can digest that sugar.

SWEATING IT OUT

You can eat all the healthy foods and avoid all the bad ones, but if you do not exercise it will not have a great effect. You need exercise to make your digestive system work right. When you exercise the body converts the food you have eaten into muscle, if you don't exercise then it will turn it into fat. Exercise has many benefits; it will burn fat, make your whole metabolism work efficiently, it will increase oxygen intake into your whole body, and it will help your body get rid of toxins.

The lack of exercise is one of the reasons why so many people get fat and sick. The body is not meant to stand still for hours on end, it was made for activity. For centuries people had to sweat and be active as part of regular life; but things have changed. Modern machines encourage inactivity. You need to take the initiative and work out on your own.

If your job is one that requires a lot of physical activity then you might be able to skip exercise or just with a little workout. Even if you have a strenuous job you can also work out those muscles that you don't use in your current job. If you walk all day long then you might need to work out on your upper muscles, and if in your job you constantly lift heavy items, you might need to work out on your legs. Round out your body this way, so that your whole body is in shape.

Of course if you are out of shape or have health problems you will need to talk to your doctor before starting exercising. If you haven't exercised in a long time, you will need to start out easy. You can not become a super athlete overnight; if you attempt to work too hard you will probably hurt yourself.

Working out doesn't have to take lots of time. In fact some people only exercise 15 minutes per day and that is all they need. If you are only trying to be healthy, and not compete in the Olympics or become a professional athlete, then you only need from 15 to 30 minutes per day. That is all you need to be healthy. Of course once you start you might like it and work out a whole hour or more everyday.

The rewards from exercise are great. You develop a toned body, your digestive system operates great, your muscles become stronger and you protect yourself against a multitude of diseases. And there is more, you live longer, and healthier. And to top it all off, your mind actually works better when you are in great physical shape. Exercise indeed is an amazing activity. So many great benefits for only a few hours invested.

Of course some people for some unknown reason have plenty of excuses for not working out. "I am too fat" Perfect you really need the exercise. "I am too tired after work" Great you really need the energy from a workout. "I don't have time", just throw that TV into the garbage can and you will have loads of time. You can keep on making excuses for not working out, but you are only deceiving yourself.

When your body is in great shape, you have an advantage over others at work. You have more natural energy than they do, and you can easily outlast them when you are in competition for a better job. You can think more clearly and faster about any problem and you mind is more alert. You can remember information better, because you can focus.

THE BEST EXERCISE

Exercise is usually divided into two types anaerobic and aerobic. Anaerobic exercise consists of low impact activities like walking. Aerobic exercise consists of heavy activity like running or weightlifting. There are many types of exercises available; and some people recommend isometrics or yoga as better alternatives to weightlifting or running.

After a lot of study of the exercise theories and ideas, I have come to the conclusion that the best exercise is a mixture of low impact anaerobic exercise with some aerobic exercise. I would suggest 80% percent anaerobic with 20 % aerobic.

The best exercise of all is simply walking; yes the oldest exercise in the world is the best exercise of all. There are many types of walking. You can walk uphill, you can walk with loads, you can speed-walk, you can march and many other variations on walking. There are whole books written on the health benefits of walking. A walk after a meal is great for the digestive process. Walking tones the whole body. It does not strain the leg muscles, causes sprains or tears. It has little impact on the whole body.

Of course I would also highly recommend swimming as a started exercise. Swimming is a non-impact exercise. Swimming exercises the whole body; it is a complete exercise that is excellent for those who are obese or overweight.

Aerobic exercise like running or weightlifting puts a tremendous strain in the body. It wears out the joints and cartilage in the body. Those exercises cause sprains, back injuries and it is just too stressful in the body. Despite all the running and muscle magazines touting the benefits of those sports, they are not the best exercises for people.

To have good health you should choose a combination of exercises that work out all the muscles in your body, in a way that put only minor strain on them. I would recommend a mixture of walking, swimming, running and weightlifting. With walking being the main part of your exercise routine.

While I advocate a little running I am not an advocate of marathon training. I think that type of training actually hurts people in the long run. And while I advocate a little weightlifting I certainly do not endorse those massive weights that frequently cause back problems and hernias in some weightlifters. I advocate moderation in running and weightlifting.

Of course if you get injured or are sick you have to adjust your exercise to match your capacity. You can not hurt your back one day and then attempt to lift 500 pounds the next day, that is just plain foolishness. If you haven't run in years, you do not suddenly sign up for a marathon. Do not get hurt by overdoing exercise.

If you are a little older you can not expect to match the strength of a young person, you have to accept that reality, but that should not stop you from doing exercise either. You can try low-stress exercise like yoga or tai chi.

REST

What does rest have to do with health? Plenty, Chronobiology (the science that studies time rhythms in nature) has discovered that our body runs on a 7-day cycle. This built in biological cycle is a way for the body to recuperate, do microscopic repairs and do preventive maintenance. That is the reason why we rest every seventh day.

Rest is also needed in between the day. Work experiments have shown that a block period of 4 work hours followed by a one hour rest period, and then 4 more work hours is the most efficient way to schedule a work day. After that time concentration diminishes dramatically and errors increase rapidly. Some people were well able to work in blocks of 5 or even 6 hours, yet the one-hour rest in between was necessary for them too.

These time cycles are natural cycles; they are part of our natural biological rhythm. Some people do not believe or respect these natural cycles. Well nature does not care whether you believe or not in its natural cycles, you will pay a price for violating your biological cycles of rest. Many religions rightly advocate that you should take one day out of seven for resting, but it doesn't matter if you are religious or not, you still need a day of rest. And you also need to rest after 4 or 5 hours of continuous activity.

Those who continuously violate these biological cycles are damaging their bodies, can't function at their prime, and are inviting a heart attack and other diseases. They are the leading cause of industrial accidents, low productivity and burn out. Furthermore they are constantly making mistakes and have to spend much time fixing their own mistakes.

Rest is not only for the body, but is also for the mind. Your mind needs to rest as surely as your body does. Actually having a rested mind is more important than having a rested body. When you leave work, forget about the job problems, stay late if you have to finish a project, but don't take work home with you.

Studying is good, but it also tires the mind. You need to rest even from studying. Let your mind rest at peace once in awhile, if you do not eventually you will be reading but retaining absolutely nothing. All that time spent studying the latest computer programs or the schoolbooks will be wasted time. Punctuate your study time with small periods of rest and switching to different subjects.

Taking a vacation is a great way to rest, but it is more than that, a vacation allows you to focus and center your body and mind. This is a time when a person unwinds from all the complexity of work. There is no such thing as a working vacation, you are either working or vacationing. Relax during the vacation, forget about the office and soak up the rest. Don't take work with you, rest and enjoy your vacation and send me a postcard.

Life is a marathon and you need the energy and stamina from rest in order to finish it. Taking the proper rest time, and recharging your body and mind is a proper use of time. This is about what is best for your mind and body. If you do not rest well you will get sick or get a heart attack and you will die.

RECREATION

Recreation is an important part of living a healthy lifestyle. You need to find ways to relax your mind and body. You have to do something that takes the stress out of your daily life. You need to do something that relaxes your body. If your job is physical then take up a hobby that will work out your mind or take a sport that will work different muscles of your body. If you work in an office then take up a vigorous sport that will work out your body or a creative art or hobby.

After work many people go home and become couch potatoes. They fail to realize that sitting down for hours watching mind numbing television is perhaps the worst form of recreation. Get rid of the sofa, throw it out on the curb and get some real recreation. The following are things that can provide recreation for your body and mind so go ahead and choose one.

SPORTS: There are hundredths of interesting sports to choose from. You can choose an intensive one like handball or an easy one like bowling. You can join a league and compete at amateur levels. Who knows you might even become good enough to compete at the professional level.

HOBBIES: You can collect stamps, seashells, toys or many other items. You can also build model cars, airplanes, tanks or even battleships. You can even enter competitions with other people in your same hobby. Gardening is a nice hobby that will also save you money in your food bill.

ARTS: You can take up painting, sculpture or photography. Some of your creations can enrich your life or even be useful items in your life. If you take up needlepoint you can make sweaters for your family, if you take up pottery you can use your pots in your cooking or for eating and drinking, maybe start a side business.

TRAVEL: You can take weekend tour and go to the beach, the parks, camping, or some tourist place. You can also explore your own city. You can visit your local places like the fire department, city hall, a factory, the court, or the police department. I am sure your city has some historical places.

SOCIAL ACTIVITIES: Perhaps you can join a local club like the elks, a veterans group, or a social action group. There are also religious groups, political groups and other interests groups. You can also volunteer in a soup kitchen, with a hospital or with another charity or social group.

SHOWS: There are many shows you can go out to watch. Maybe you can go to the opera, the theater or a skating show. At least go to the movies. You can also go to those places where they have a show and a meal, places like medieval times or the circus. Check your area for things like carnivals, fairs and parades, and you will find some of those.

THERE IS NO REASON TO BECOME A COUCH POTATO!

CLEANLINESS

Cleanliness is a key component of health. You need to wash or clean yourself in order to remain healthy. When your body sweats it gets rid of toxins and salts in your body. Those substances accumulated on the skin of the body and they will eventually start decaying and putrefying, and you will start to smell bad. Use a brush or something that will actually remove dead skin from your body instead of a flimsy cotton towel.

One of the big problems in modern life is that water is often chlorinated to kill germs, which is a good thing, but the bad thing is that they leave the chlorine in and that is bad. Your body will absorb the chlorine through the skin, and you will also get it in the steam if you take hot showers. Chlorine is a dangerous poison; it is deadly to humans too. The best solution is to get a shower filter, yes they do make those for people who want to shower in clean water, get one and you will have healthy skin.

But cleanliness is more than simply taking a shower. It also includes brushing your teeth, cleaning your nails, and washing your hands before touching any food. You also have to wear clean clothes. It also includes your house and your work area. Dirt and trash create fouls smells, vermin infestation and disease. It doesn't matter how poor you are; a bar of soap is still the cheapest thing around. You can take many other steps to be clean.

Of course do not forget to clean those areas that are often neglected by others, I am talking about between the toes, behind the ears, and inside the ears. The nostrils can also be cleansed from all dirt, and lets us not forget to brush the tongue once in a while. Yes these areas and others need to be cleaned once in a while.

Yes doing all these things for cleanliness takes a little time, yet it is well-invested time. Being clean is more than a matter of health but also of image and social graces. People who smell bad will have social problems with family, friends, and strangers; no one wants to be around a funky smelling stinking person.

Uncleanness will produce sickness in your person and will also affect those around you. When you are sick your family will have to take care of you, and you will miss days from work. In the course of the day you might get a little dirty, especially if you work outdoors, yet during your lunch time, you can take a few minutes to at least clean up a little and wash your hands and wash your face, before eating.

The best way to have things clean is to keep them that way. If you will engage in an activity that might produce dirt then put old newspapers, cardboard or towels on the floor area so that when you finish, you can quickly clean up your area. Clean your dirty hands before you handle any food. You may need to wear an apron or protective clothing. Remember it is easier to keep things clean than to clean them afterwards.

Yes, you do need to put in a little effort to clean up and then keep clean your person, your house, and your items; for filth brings sickness and disease. Cleaning up does take some time and effort but it is a needed and healthful activity.

MENTAL HEALTH

Your mental health is very important in order to have a good and successful life. With a damaged mind you will live a very miserable existence. You need to care for the well being of your mind. There are plenty of things that you can do for your mental health. People who develop mental problems have often contributed to their own problems.

EMOTIONS: It is estimated that half of all the diseases are caused by internal emotions. Bad feelings like hatred, anger, fear, guilt, bitterness and other similar emotions cause or aggravate many physical diseases and also create mental disturbances. They can cause a person to have an emotional breakdown and even go so far as to cause madness.

HABITS: Drugs, alcohol, tobacco, caffeine and even sugar affect the mind. These bad substances create a devastating toll on our brains. The mind becomes altered and becomes addicted to the soothing effects of all these drugs. There comes a point when people become unable to function without a dose of these harmful substances.

LIFESTYLE: The activities you participate in will affect your mind. Many people suffer from irritation, lack of concentration, nervousness and other psychotic anomalies because of the lifestyle they lead. If you skip sleep, or have erratic sleeping patterns your mind will be affected. Going to too many parties will take a toll on your mindset.

DIET: Believe it or not, but your diet does affect your mind. What you eat becomes chemicals that reach your brain. If you eat a bad diet you will feel weak not only in your body but also in your mind. There are foods, like vegetables, fruits and grains that will keep your mind alert and focused. Greasy meats tend to make you sleepy and tired.

REST: The mind needs to rest too. There are times when you should lay down your problems and worries and just relax. Take some time to just lie down and look at the clouds or look at a beautiful sunset. Stop thinking and just soak up the world. Go and have a relaxing vacation and forget about work, problems and worries.

MEDITATION: Meditation does not have to be done by using yoga and chanting mindless mantras or slogans. Mediation is simply relaxing your mind and think about good things. It is also about calmly thinking about what you have in life, Think about your spouse, children, friends, and all the good things you have in your life.

EXERCISE: Many people are not aware that the mind also needs exercise, yes it does. Just how does a person exercise his mind? By giving it hard problems to solve. Or by solving jigsaw or crossword puzzles, riddles, cryptograms and word searches. A fun way is to play games like chess, mahjong; boggle, scrabble or memory tiles.

Your mind is a marvelous and incredible creation. It was created to process information, but for that to happen; you need to give it information to process. Read good books or magazines, listen to tapes, and take trips. You need to take care of you mind or else it will be gone and once it is gone it is very hard to get it back.

FEEDING YOUR MIND

You have a marvelous mind and it is up to you to treat it right and feed it right. Whatever you feed your mind is what you will become. Health starts in the mind. If you sow in your mind negativity and a sour attitude; that is exactly what you'll reap in your body. Instead read, listen and think of those things, which are positive, outstanding and great. Strengthen your mind with good ideas and you will reap a healthier body.

Don't dwell on personal problems. Listen buddy, everybody has problems; people are born to trouble as the sparks fly upward. Hashing and rehashing your problems in your mind will not solve them; and you can become physically sick by obsessive worry about your problems, thus creating more problems. If you have problems instead of worrying about them; you have to take proactive action to resolve them.

Avoid the bad news. There is nothing wrong with keeping informed however you must realize that the negative, bad and abnormal is what gets publicized, but the good gets ignored. All those bad news only tend to mess with your mental and emotional state and raise your blood pressure. If you still want to read the news, then get a weekly magazine or wait till later in the day. Avoid critical and negative articles or commentaries.

Avoid stressful programs. What you watch has a tremendous effect on your mind and health. If you watch a lot of horror or violent programs it will have a harmful effect on your body, also avoid listening to shock radio and shock TV. Everything that arouses your emotions and makes you angry or upset will affect your mind and body.

Run away from the gloom and doom types. There are some people who only talk about the bad things of this world. Yes the world has problems, but no the world is not ending tomorrow. Bad things have happened, are happening and will continue to happen, but humanity will just keep on moving. Fear will cause many health problems.

Avoid controversies. Politics and religions are bound to create controversy, which might degenerate into ideological wars. Yes they are important to many people, but tact and consideration should be used when discussing these subjects. Arguing is a waste of time and counterproductive. No argument has ever convinced a person who is not open minded.

Think on these things. Whatsoever is true, whatsoever is honest, whatsoever is just, whatsoever is pure, whatsoever is lovely, whatsoever is good news, if there be any virtue, if there be any praise, think on these things.

If you feed your mind with bad ideas and thoughts these items you will be in constant anger and your blood pressure will shoot sky-high. You have to feed your mind on the good things of life, focus on positive events, positive people, and positive actions. The choice of what you feed your mind is solely yours.

READ GOOD STORIES. Feed your mind on the many good classics, also read the uplifting stories about people who faced adversity and triumphed, people who made great deeds for the good of humanity. Relax and learn that despite any problems or tragedies humanity will keep on pushing forward toward better things.

MIND CARE

Your mind is the most important possession you have. There are plenty of people in mental hospitals or walking around who have lost theirs. How do you keep your mind healthy? Just what steps can you take to keep your mind in top shape? Fortunately there are plenty of things you can do to take care of your mind.

DON'T DO DRUGS. Avoid illegal drugs, they are mind altering. They will physically change your mind and will destroy your ability to learn or reason and make good decisions. Drug addicts behave in irrational ways.

DON'T DRINK ALCOHOL. It is a mind-altering substance just like a drug. It might not be as harmful as an illegal drug, but it does destroy some neurons. A little bit of alcohol can relax you but it also tends to lower your inhibitions.

DON'T SMOKE. Tobacco has many toxic substances that reach the mind and produce a calming effect. It gives a sense of pleasure and is highly addictive. It alters the personality and creates a hardening of attitude.

GO EASY ON THE SUGAR: Sugar tends to create a euphoric state of mind. It does it by releasing endorphins in the mind. It is highly addictive and if used in excess creates behavioral and hyperactivity problems.

AVOID TOXIC SUBSTANCES: Many of today's cleaning chemicals are toxic to the mind; it also goes for many other substances like paints, and glues. Use face filters whenever using any of these toxic substances.

EAT HEALTHY FOOD: Everything that you eat affects your mind too. Once food reaches the stomach it gets broken down into its basic chemical components. And those substances travel through bloodstream into the mind.

HAVE MENTAL TESTS: There are some tests that can be made to check your mental ability and any abnormalities. Taking care of your mental health is just like taking care of your body, do it at least once per year.

TAKE SUPPLEMENTS: There are some supplements that appear to have some positive effect on the mind, although nothing has been proven conclusively. The most popular are Ginkgo Biloba, vitamins E, B, lecithin, curcumin and others.

CONTROL YOU MIND: Learn to focus your mind on ideas or thoughts. You have to be able to direct your mind instead of letting it wander off in different wild tangents. You have to control your mind and guided it in any direction you want.

BE AWARE: If you suddenly develop a mental problem, do not put it off, you need to check into it as soon as possible. You wouldn't continue driving with a flat tire, isn't your mind more precious than a car?

GOOD EMOTIONS

Everyone has emotions, but being highly emotional will hurt your body. You will be on a roller coaster of hormonal instability. You will be up and down so many times your whole system will be out of whack. Your blood pressure will shoot up and your ulcers will start acting up. It is pointless to take medicine for some diseases, because your problem is not physical but emotional, and until you learn to control your emotions, you won't be healed.

You have to take control of your emotions, so that your body is not adversely affected. Now don't get me wrong and think that I am saying you should be a robot, that is not what I am saying for emotions is what makes us humans, what I am saying is that you should ride your emotions instead of your emotions riding you.

There are some emotions that are actually are beneficial to our health. Your goal should be to have more of the good emotions and less of the bad emotions. The positive emotions are love, sympathy, generosity, compassion, humility and other similar ones. These good emotions release endorphins, which make us feel good and help to heal the body. That warm feeling you have when you love someone is produced by endorphins released from your brain.

Seek to always be in a positive state so that your health will improve. Be around those people who make you feel good and do those things that uplift your spirit. See and read those things that arouse good feelings. If something good has happened (like you got a raise) then go ahead and enjoy it. There is absolutely nothing wrong with feeling happy and enjoying life. Celebrate the good things in life, and be happy.

One of the best emotions for healing is happiness, learn to laugh and enjoy life, get a bunch of funny comic books and learn to laugh. Laughter does good like if it was a medicine. It takes away depression and worries out of your mind. Get some of the old comedy shows that have become classics.

Love people, love your life, love is the supreme emotion. If you learn to love yourself and your life you will heal much faster. The fastest way to love yourself is to do good deeds for others, it is a circle of love, you give love to others and they will give love back to you, try it, it works.

Be at peace with yourself and others learn to forgive and forget, let go of all grudges, understand that all humans make mistakes and are flawed. Be kind and patience with those who in ignorance or because of some character flaw hurt you a long ago. You be the bigger person and take the first step toward reconciliation.

There is nothing wrong with having or showing emotions, but keep them under control or else your health will suffer. Good emotions will heal you so seek for them, yes there will still be problems and difficulties in life, but if you have a sense of humor you will be able to handle them a lot better.

SLEEP SWEET SLEEP

Sleep is a part of our biological cycle. The sleep cycle of 8/16 hours comes out to one hour of sleep for every two hours awake. The average sleep time is eight hours, some needing more and others needing less. The sleep cycle has five stages, that is why it is important that the sleep time be continuous otherwise these stages get interrupted. In old times most people went to sleep after dark, but modern times have disrupted the cycle.

The problem is that not everyone sleeps right. Too many people are walking around half-asleep, causing traffic accidents and work accidents. Too many people can't concentrate on the job right; because they are sleep deprived or they have erratic sleep patterns. They are walking zombies, only kept awake by harmful caffeine.

Caffeine is perhaps the worst enemy of sleep. Unfortunately we drink and eat an abundance of caffeine. It is in coffee, in sodas, in teas and in chocolate. After a day at the office swallowing all those cups of coffee it is not wonder many people have trouble falling asleep. Caffeine will jolt you and wake you up but at a high cost.

Truck drivers are notorious for falling asleep at the wheel, in an effort to spend more time at the wheel; they sleep few hours and take caffeine by the buckets. Laws have been passed to regulate the amount of hours a truck driver can work, but that has not helped some to get good sleeping habits.

The other big problem is the over-excitement we get from the entertainment industry. We love to see scary or violent movies. We love roller coasters, car races, sports and games. We watch newscasts full of car chases and dangerous events. We are adrenaline junkies. Is it any wonder we have trouble sleeping when our mind is over-stimulated?

One of the worst innovations created is the third shift, commonly known as the "graveyard". There is a very good reason why it is nicknamed like that. It will send people to their early grave. The night was made for sleeping, not working.

Then when we have trouble falling asleep how do we remedy it? Well we take sleeping pills. What a horrible solution! Those sleeping pills disrupt the normal sleeping habits and make many drug-dependent. Not to mention the possible harmful effects on the mind, like hallucinations and nightmares. Don't even think about taking sleeping pills.

If you have problems sleeping or you feel sleepy after lunch then you need to get control of your sleep. Try taking some of the following steps. First get rid of caffeine in your diet. Then establish a sleep time and a wake up time; make sure to stick to your sleep schedule. Also avoid watching so much TV, for it stimulates your mind. You can also do some light physical exercise a few minutes before going to sleep.

If all these steps do not help you then you could take some herbal teas like chamomile or valerian. As a last resort go see a naturopath, for you probably have some disease that needs to be taken care of.

THE ENVIRONMENT

The environment that you live on determines a lot of your health. If you live in a place that is polluted by chemicals or live in an electronic cottage, then you are bound to have many health problems. The same goes for a home where trash is everywhere or other hazards exist. What can you do about it? You can move to a place that is not polluted or you can clean up your place.

It would be great if we could move to another planet that is not polluted and start over but we can not do that. So if you are not able to move to a less polluted area, you still can take action. You can help by volunteering to clean your community. A healthy community has less sick people overall. Every activity you participate to help your community; helps you too.

Besides local community involvement what else can you do? Well you can take some actions to make your home a safer and healthier place. The number of things you can check for and actions you take are many, but you have to start one thing at a time.

You could start by making sure that your house paint does not contain lead. This is a dangerous element that causes many health problems. You can also make sure that you do not have any asbestos. Check your house for any other dangerous building material and replace it with something less toxic.

Then check you house for electrical problems, the numbers of houses with electrical problems are many. This includes checking for shorts, wrong polarization, and excessive EMF output. When you have too many electrical gadgets turned, your house becomes an electronic danger to your health.

Then check all your property for any contamination or dangerous chemicals and clean it up or remove it. There are some people who have a lot of illness that arise from the house or property they live in. They keep on wondering why they get sick so often without realizing that a sick house makes its inhabitants sick.

How clean is your house, could it pass a health inspection? Do you have toxic materials all over you house? You could be breathing toxic fumes from all the products that are in your house. How is your ventilation system? Are you breathing clean or polluted air? Do you have any gas leaks that are slowly making you sick?

We have a lot of technology to make our house environment cleaner. Some people buy air purifiers and humidifiers, others buys some other gadgets, however I believe the answer is not more technology but less. There are plenty of steps you can take to make your home healthier for you; all it takes is a little imagination.

How about having some indoor plants to give you fresh oxygen. How about having a house with lots of big windows to let the sunshine in. How about avoiding using harmful pesticides in the garden or the grass. How about planting some nice big trees that will give you nice shade and fresh clean oxygen.

PART III: WARNINGS & RANTS

MERCHANTS OF DEATH

I really don't know where to start, because there so much to say and all of it is bad. First of all I will not shout or even insinuate that the food merchants and others that I name here are evil people. I am sure most of them are pretty decent folk, who probably have a nice family and think they are doing a service with their business. I am not seeking to besmirch their character, I am positive that most are fine church going people.

The point I am trying to make is not about some evil corporation or evil masterminds. The point I am making is that there is a lot of ignorance, naiveté and foolishness in the food industry. Every one of these merchants sell products that harm our health and produce death, they are definitely merchants of death. I am sure they would defend themselves and their products with all their means as beneficial, but the reality is that they are bringers of disease and death.

The number one spot in my book has to be the fast food purveyors. There is absolutely nothing healthy about eating in fast food joints. They are death traps, literally. I may be offending a trillion dollar industry, but sincerely I do not care. Their food is deadly to our health; they are killing people with their junk. The only reason you should go into a fast food restaurant is if you have a death wish. I am not only talking about hamburger chains, but I include all other fast food chains there are. I am sure that someone will point to me one or two places that offer good healthy food, but those exceptions are few, I am talking about the 95 percent of the industry.

Number two, following real close to number one, are the processed food industries. In the name of profit they add sugar, fat and salt to most of their products. They need to add those otherwise they would not sell as much. Of course they can get away with it, because the public keeps on buying their delicious products never mind that those products are harmful. And I did not even mention the harm caused by the way they manufacture, process and preserve the foods they sell. They are really killing people, and it is all done in the pursuit of profit.

Who is next? They would have to be the meat industry. They are selling us 'aged" meat that should not be eaten. The animals are loaded with growth hormones and never allowed to exercise. Then when the animals get sick because of the conditions they are kept in, they are shot full of antibiotics, which then are passed on to us. I shall not even go into the horrors of adding nitrates and nitrites to cured meat. There is so much more that could be said about the meat industry but you should get the idea.

OK, next one. I just can not let big farms of the hook; they basically are destroying the goodness in vegetables and fruits. They genetically modify produce in order to make it more resistant to disease and more productive. They are changing the nature of produce into something that is not the way nature intended. Then to make matters worse, they add artificial fertilizers, and then pesticides. Pesticides serve only one purpose, and that is to kill. You hear that, pesticides are poisons that kill, and you are eating them in your salads.

Of course let us not forget the chemical industry. This industry is poisoning people, animals, plants and the planet. The chemical industry has so much death and blood in its hands that none of their chemical cleansers can clean it up. We eat preservatives and additives in our foods, and we also absorb them in our skin as deodorants, shampoos, lotions, creams and perfumes. Also all the cleaners, household products eventually end up in the food chain and we end up eating them.

Listen up people, the food merchants are selling us death, and it is all being done in the name of profit. Can foods be produced naturally? Yes they can, but the profits are not as big as using artificial means. All the chemicals used to keep the foods from spoiling are killing us. The people who rule the food chain supply want to make big profits, and your health is not a concern. Of course if a product caused instant death it would raise a big ruckus and be withdrawn, but no one seems to mind a slow poisoning.

NUTRITION NUTS

Nutrition is a very important subject but we need to be aware of some problems and dangers. We need to understand that just like in any field, whether it is law or medicine; there are incompetent practitioners who really are not qualified to practice and also charlatans taking advantage of people, and of course some that are mentally unstable.

Some nutritionists or organizations will promote this or that product as a miracle food, and of course they often just happen to sell the product. Any claim that is too good to be believed is probably a sham. Of course some people sincerely believe in the power of what they peddle. Their sincerity or passion for their products does not make their products any more effective.

Of course everyone in the world needs calcium or some other nutrient in the body, but they do not have to buy the special formula patented by so and so person or company. Of course everyone can benefit from this or that product, but humanity has managed to live for thousands of years without the latest invention.

No I will not endorse anyone's products or formulas, I am not a pitchman for any organization, I do not care if their products are truly beneficial or not. My aim is to inform people about the need for vitamin C, not that they have to buy someone's formula of vitamin C and that only a special formula will work miracles in your body. Sorry but I do not promote miracle formulas, so do not even send me any offers, I am not for sale, I only promote good health and information that will generate good health.

Now regarding natural foods; first of all there is no fruit, vegetable or bread that will give all the nutrients that your body needs. You need to eat a variety of natural foods to maintain good health. There is no miracle bread or food that will keep you healthy by itself. All those miracle foods are nothing but a sophisticated scam, yet people keep on falling for them.

Despite all the wild claims of some vegetarians meat has not proven to be bad for you, only the excessive eating of meat causes health problems. The same goes for milk and cheese. For thousands of years people in different cultures have eaten meat, eggs, milk and cheese as part of their diets with no harmful effects to their bodies. But of course these people ate organic meat and organic dairy products.

Now let us talk about vitamins, and minerals. You do need vitamins, minerals and other nutrients and of course the vitamin merchants want you to buy their products. The truth is that you get most of your vitamins and minerals from the foods that you eat. As long as you eat nutritious foods you do not need to buy any pills, liquids or whatever.

Now regarding nutritional supplements, a lot of them are just hype. They make wild and exaggerated claims that they can provide nutrition and make you lose weight. Well this is usually jus a sophisticated scam. There is nothing wrong with taking nutritional supplements for your health, but it would be cheaper, better and healthier if you ate the natural foods the supplements are extracted from.

Let me repeat again, that if you eat nutritious foods you do not need any vitamins, minerals, nutritional supplements or any thing else. Let's get real; if you eat a horrible diet those products are not going to make up for the deficiencies. You can not, I repeat you can not, make up for a horrible diet by taking anything; it just doesn't work that way. Perhaps I have offended the vitamin and supplement vendors, but sincerely these merchants are selling products that are really not needed.

If you are not sure you eat a varied nutritious diet or maybe you want to ensure that you get all the vitamins and minerals that you need, then go ahead and compare the different products in the market and buy those that have what you need. Buy good quality vitamins from reputable companies not those cheap bargains which are made with the cheapest materials available.

Beware of those who peddle a strange natural food as a super-food that will keep you healthy and make you live a hundred years, you can bet it is a scam. There is nothing wrong with eating nuts for your nutrition, they are good and healthy, but you should be wary of listening to nutrition nuts, they could seriously harm your health.

THE DECEIVERS

Advertisers are in the business of promoting the products of their customers. They are paid to increase the amount of sales of x product; that is their whole purpose. They will advertise using every trick in the book and creating new ones. They are masters at the art of deception and persuasion. Wake up and refuse to be taken in by their slick advertising. They will advertise cleverly to whatever demographic is their primary target.

If the product is harmful or even kills people it is none of their concern. They are not in the business of educating people or promoting the health of the people. They have zero obligation to look out for the welfare of the public. You have to realize that the only purpose of commercials and advertisements is to make you desire and buy the product they are drumming.

Businesspeople are in the business of making money. Some take this so far as to sell whatever people want regardless of the consequences. There have been plenty of deadly products advertised as healthful, until the product starts hurting or even killing people. Then the product is withdrawn, but by then it is too late for some people.

The tobacco and alcohol pushers think of themselves as decent law abiding folk, yet their products kill thousands of people every year. The sugar industry and the food conglomerates must think of themselves as decent people, without thinking that their unhealthful products cause much misery and suffering.

Of course every business industry will fight any attempt to regulate their products or any bad publicity of their products. It is only natural for they are protecting their livelihood. Wars have been fought to protect the trade of harmful products. The English fought against China over opium. Loggers will fight environmentalists over trees.

The industries will fight in many ways to protect their products. They will use laws and influence to pass legislation beneficial to them. They will seek ways to discredit the critics of their products. They might fund studies, which show their products in a good light. They will do whatever is legal and maybe semi-legal to protect their self-interest.

If you want to be healthy you have to realize that you have to decide to think for yourself, and don't be swayed by commercials and advertisements which use many clever mind tricks and twisting of the truth. They are experts at using emotional and sentimental tricks to get you to buy their products. You have to learn to be independent in your thoughts.

You might also have to fight the mockery or fun of other people who make fun of those who care about their own health. Some might think you are a little crazy for caring about your health, but the really crazy thing is not to care about your health. Some may tempt you or try to sabotage your efforts out of ignorance or even out of ulterior motives.

The whole point is that living a healthy lifestyle will require you to be a very independent thinking person. You have to think about what is good for you health, not what is good for the pocketbook of some businessmen. Living a healthy life is not the easy way.

DEADLY MEDICINE

The pharmaceutical industries (Big Pharma) will hate me for what I am about to say, but since I have offended just about every multi-billion dollar industry, I am not about to let them get away without a scratch. To me they are just drug pushers using slick TV commercials and every other medium possible to get you hooked in their drugs.

Big Pharma is just another industry out to make a quick buck. They are selling you a big pack of lies in those drugs. Their drugs are often dangerous, some are actually deadly. Their drugs, which are supposed to heal people actually kill thousands of people every year, those people don't die from a disease but from a reaction to the medical drugs. You can check the statistics.

How can Big Pharma get away with it? Simple they contribute millions of dollars to politicians; that is why some of their drugs get approval by the FDA. Of course there are studies on the drugs, but who is conducting those studies? Labs that have a lot to gain conduct most of those studies; they are basically scientists for sale.

Would the FDA the agency responsible for safeguarding the health of the public approve a harmful drug? Come on get serious, harmful drugs have routinely been approved to be later recalled when people start dying. Of course there are denials, lawsuits and penalties, but those are just considered as regular costs of the drug industry. A little of the profits are forked over and the cycle starts over again.

Hear this **no drug can heal you of any disease**. You can not be healed by any drug of anything. Only your body can heal you. Your body has a self-healing mechanism that will heal you. Most of their drugs actually interfere with this natural healing process and make it even harder for the body to heal, so you stay dependent on drugs even more.

If no drug can heal of anything, then why do people take them? Because drugs take away the symptoms of the disease. Listen, pain is not a sickness; pain is an alarm that tells you there is a problem with your body. A pain reliever will take away the pain, but the cause of the pain still in the body. It is like disconnecting a fire alarm to a house that is burning. The house still slowly burning but there is no longer an alarm telling you that it is burning. Wake up people and understand that drugs take away the symptoms but not the disease, the disease still down there smoldering slowly and destroying your body.

The silliest and most profitable new money making scheme by the drug industry is the new drugs that take away the side effects of the other drugs. Since all drugs give side effects someone in the industry decided that they could also make money from that problem. So now there is a more profitable vicious circle. A person takes a drug for a disease; then takes another drug to get rid of the side effects of the first drug, and then takes still another drug to get rid of the side effects of the second drug. Oh man, what a marvelous way to make a fortune from the suckers.

Of course the drug industry hates competition, which is why they have invested millions of dollars discrediting and even outlawing herbal medicines under the guise of safety. Herbal medicines have a better track record than drugs, but results do not matter when there are powerful financial interests.

I do not want to have an army of BIG Pharma lawyers knocking at my door, so everything that I have said here is simply my humble opinion; after all I still have freedom of expression and really what have they to fear from me, I do not have any millions of dollars to advertise the truth, like they do their lies. Listen, Big Pharma is simply selling deadly medicine; don't fall for their deceptive advertising. I really don't care about their drugs; I do not risk my life to make Big Pharma richer. I do not take any of their dangerous medicines. Why, because their medicines only mask the symptoms or make the disease worse, they do not take care of the cause of the disease.

How can I even say that? First because this is a free country where people are free to express their opinion. Plenty of people including myself have refused to take drugs and have treated all of our diseases using herbal medicine. I have realized that those expensive drugs instead of healing only make the sickness even worse. Many people have been on dangerous drugs for years without ever been healed, it is only when they switched to herbs that they finally were healed.

There are many thousands of people who have forsaken drugs and tried natural medicine and have gotten better results than by using drugs. Of course the drugs companies try to silence the voice of these people, but the truth can not remain hidden for ever. Natural medicine does not have the harmful side effects of drugs, but of course even using natural medicine requires the right knowledge in order to use it properly.

RACING TOWARD OBLIVION

If everything that we did only affected us, then I would say that we deserve all the disease and sickness that this modern society has. All our problems are self-earned. We are only sowing what we have reaped. But it is not just us everything that we are doing now will affect generations to come.

The oceans and the rivers were truly bountiful with plenty of fish and medicinal products for our healing. Fish are excellent, good tasting and nutritious. They have plenty of protein and omega oils. Whole cultures had lived on sea products for generations and enjoyed excellent health. Unfortunately we begun to mechanize the ocean and overfishing depleted the oceans, not to mention all the pollution and mercury poisoning we have done.

It was not enough that we planted and harvested fruits and vegetables from nature; we begun to modified our foods, we begun with artificial fertilizers and pesticides. Now we are bent on destroying our food thru genetically modified foods, and of course let us not forget about the radiation of food. Talk about being foolish and crazy.

Once we destroy all the food in our oceans and in nature what will we eat? What will our children eat? That is if we can even have any more children.

We willingly eat and drink artificial foods that give zero nutrition; we willingly put on chemicals in our bodies in an effort to hide our human odors. We take all kinds of drugs illegal and medical and we dare to think they won't have any impact on our descendents? We are putting things in our bodies that will make us sterile and cause weakness and deformities in our children.

Nature is wonderful it has provided us with everything that we need to thrive; unfortunately we just can't leave things alone. We seem to have a destructive gene that seeks to destroy what nature has created for us. We love to tinker with things until we totally foul things up. What is worst now we have begun to thinker with the human DNA, does anyone seriously think we are going to do any better in this new field?

We indiscriminately give antibiotics to every animal that we farm. And then we shoot ourselves with more antibiotics. Come on stop this craziness. We are just making sure that the antibiotics will not be any longer effective by creating super bugs. Then what are we going to do? What will our children do when they realize that we got the benefits of antibiotics, but all they have are super bugs to deal with?

We pollute the air, the water and the ground. We pave over good farming land and dump our waste all over nature. But it seems to us that simply destroying nature is not enough for us. Now we are engaged in a race to destroy our own children's future. What are we going to leave our children? A polluted world, an uninhabitable planet? A trillion dollar debt? Are we going to leave our children a world where there is no real food and they will have no clean breathable air? Do we even care?

PART IV: SOME SOLUTIONS

NATURAL HEALING

The best thing is to never get sick. If you eat nutritious foods and take good care of your body and don't engage in bad habits or a harmful lifestyle you will have a lot less diseases than others, but not matter how much care we take sometimes disease still strikes. When that happens, then a little knowledge goes a long way.

When disease comes natural medicine is the best way to go. Nature's plants and herbs are not as harmful as medical drugs. Natural medicines have been used for centuries and have been successful in treating many diseases. Of course I can not recommend any natural medicine for any disease because I could be prosecuted for practicing medicine without a degree, but I can tell you the truth, and they can not stop me from doing that.

Recently there has been a push by the drug industry to silence anyone advocating natural medicine or bad mouthing the deadly drug industry. Why? Because natural medicine is not patentable and they can not make money of it. The war against natural medicine is at an all time high. They send outrageously threatening letters and massive multi-million dollar advertising campaigns to discredit natural medicine.

Big Pharma has the money to hire the best spoke persons and use ever trick clean and dirty to make natural medicine seem ineffective or even dangerous. And of course they use the FDA as their lapdog to hunt and harass anyone advocating the use of natural medicine.

Listen, natural medicines and herbs are not dangerous if used properly. And yes they are effective if used correctly. Natural medicine works slower than drugs, but there is no risk of side effects. One of the big lies by Big Pharma is that natural herbs do not give precise doses like their drugs do. That is a bunch of crock; the body will take the needed amount of ingredients from natural herbs and discard the rest. That is why we have an efficient elimination system. Of course any herb or drug if taken in excessive doses could be toxic.

Many natural herbs are better than drugs and the drug companies often know it, but of course the medical establishment will never tell you that. Why admit the truth if doing so will hurt your bottom line.

Natural medicine has been used for centuries for healing. It has been used in every culture. Even in the bible we find some prophets of God who used natural healing. Of course before using herbs see an experienced herbalist who understands which herbs are right for which disease and in what amounts.

Besides herbs what are some other natural medicines? There are many, some of them have been used in many cultures around the world. There are body cleanses, fruits and vegetables diet, fasting, hydrotherapy, tonics, oxygen cleanses and many others.

The body cleanses are very popular, there are different kinds; there is colon cleansing, candida cleansing, and many other types. Usually a person is given some herbs or natural products in order to cause the body cleansing. The fruit and vegetable diet is where a person only eats raw fruits and vegetables for a certain amount of time. Fasting is a biblical custom where a person doesn't eat for a certain amount of time.

There is hydrotherapy. This is the method where pure water is used to treat disease. The person drinks water to purify the body and bathes in pure water to cleanse the system.

Oxygen healing is where a person goes high into a mountain and practices breathing exercises. By breathing oxygen deeply the person cleanses the system from impurities. The person does this for about thirty days in order to cleanse the system.

Natural healing techniques are better and more successful than dangerous drugs, and are able to heal most diseases even cancer, Yes even cancer!

NATURAL REMEDIES

Natural remedies can be done using herbs, plants, animal and mineral products. These can help ameliorate a disease, prevent it or even cure it, but this requires a naturopath who has studied natural medicine for years.

Herbal remedies have been used for centuries and continue to be used in every country for diseases and healing. The reason they are used is because they work, are cheaper, and have few side effects. Some problems do develop when people take herbal remedies without knowing their proper use.

Many doctors will not prescribe any herbal remedies, because they don't know anything about them or they get bonuses if they prescribe drugs. So if you tell your doctor that you are using a natural herb that ignorance will usually lead that doctor to be skeptical or worried about your decision.

Despite all the millions of dollars in smear campaigns against herbal remedies, they keep on going strong. People are not that stupid as to believe all the propaganda from the pharmaceutical companies. People do know that herbs are better than drugs.

Natural medicine contain a number of chemicals that are in balance and those chemicals working together in combination are able to heal while at the same time counteract any potential side effects.

Of course this raises another problem. There are lots of charlatans making money of people selling herbs. These scam artists take advantage of the ignorance of people and sell herbs about which they know nothing about. The problem with this is that there are not authoritative bodies to license herbalists. It would be great if herbalists were required at least four years of botanical and medical studies before allowed to sell or recommend anything to the public.

Another thing to keep in mind is that no herb or plant can heal all diseases. The reason is simple; every disease has a different cause. The plant or herb that can "cure it all" does not exist. Anyone who tells people that a certain herb, tea or potion can heal all diseases is perpetrating a scam upon the ignorant and the gullible.

Herbal teas are a great way to heal some diseases, those made with fresh leaves work the best. Some herbs or herbal oils are excellent when used externally. Others can be used as vapors that you can smell.

Another way to use natural medicine is in combination. There are certain plants than when used in the right combinations produce a powerful effect. Of course let us not forget the other natural medicines like animal products and natural minerals. Properly used these too can help in the healing of diseases.

YOUR AMAZING HEALING POWERS

Your body has amazing healing powers. When you cut a finger the body will mobilize and heal the wound. When you break a bone it will heal and restore even stronger than before. There have been cases where a damaged brain has rerouted itself to avoid damaged areas and some parts of the brain have assumed other functions. And all of this is done by the body on its own wisdom, without any outside intervention.

Your body has an amazing self-healing mechanism. It can heal almost any damaged part of itself. And when it can not heal a part, it finds a way to compensate for the damaged part. Many times the body compensates for a disability by sharpening the other senses. It is well known that deaf people learn to compensate for their disability by developing more sensibility in their other senses.

We are just beginning to understand this self-healing mechanism. Many people have been able to activate this self-healing mechanism and recover from devastating diseases. Some of the healings have been so fast they seem almost miraculous. Others have occurred so completely that few believe the person healed was ever seriously sick at all.

If you are sick you can get healed from just about any disease by activating this self-healing mechanism the difficult part is to find out how to activate it. Some are able to activate their healing mechanism easily while others have a hard time doing it. Some by using one technique while others by using a completely different approach.

The issue is that although every person has a self-healing mechanism not every one has an efficient self-healing mechanism. Some people have abused their body to the point that this mechanism is barely able to function at all. The lifestyle you lead can severely damage your healing mechanism. If you work without resting, and go to sleep late at nigh and live on junk food, you are slowly destroying your healing mechanism.

When your healing mechanism is damaged, you have to find a way to restore it. You could start with the physical disciplines, like changing your nutrition first. If that doesn't do the trick, you could try herbal medicines. Maybe extra doses of vitamins, tonics or juicing might do the trick. You could keep on going down the line by trying acupuncture, deep massage, steam therapy and many other techniques until you find something that clicks.

Perhaps the problem can be fixed by using mental disciplines. You could try developing a mental positive attitude. You could try releasing your anger and other bad feelings. You could try self-talk healing phrases. You could try any of the different number of mental disciplines like prayer or meditation.

The whole point is to keep on trying till you find the method that works. Perhaps you could try a multi-pronged approach where you practice many healing disciplines. One of them is bound to reactivate your healing mechanism or perhaps a combination of them could do it. Don't give up; your body is a wondrous machine capable of performing miraculous cures.

CURING ALL DISEASES

All diseases are curable; there is no single disease that is not curable. Yes cancer is curable; any and all types of cancers are curable. Yes diabetes is curable, so is hypertension and every single other disease. Any person who says there is no cure for this or that disease is a fool or ignorant. My advice is to turn around and run far away from that person.

If all diseases are curable then why are they not cured? Because of many factors, one of them is simple ignorance. For instance for many years sailors died from scurvy when all that was needed to cure it was vitamin C, which is in oranges and limes. A British doctor discovered that the cure was available all along. After that the British navy always carried oranges or lemons in their cargo.

There are many other stories of people dying for centuries of diseases that are now easily cured. It wasn't that the disease was incurable; it was that they simple did not know how to cure it. The same happens today, there is widespread ignorance about curing some new diseases, but I would bet that the cure is probably right there in front of us.

Another powerful reason diseases are not cured is because there are powerful interests which have a lot invested in the continuation of diseases. Think about this all the people working for those medical associations like the cancer societies who would be out of business if the disease were suddenly wiped out. The same would happen to the arthritis foundations and the diabetic institutes.

There is a strong incentive not to cure any disease; the money is not in curing diseases but in managing them. Most modern medicine is moving away from finding a cure for any disease and instead they have moved toward the management of disease. The whole diabetic care system is geared toward managing the disease while finding a cure is not longer the goal; that is why anyone even mentioning a cure for diabetes is labeled or considered a heretic, a charlatan or a simple ignorant fellow. Powerful interests are in the way of finding any cure for diabetes. A cure would destroy a multi-million dollar business and that is something those profiting from diabetes do not want to happen.

Perhaps the biggest opponent of finding a real cure for any disease is the Pharmaceutical industry also known as Big Pharma. The moment a person is cured then that person no longer needs their dangerous drugs. That is why Big Pharma will pour billions into the management of disease but not a single penny toward finding a permanent cure for any disease. If you see their television adds not one of their drugs promises to cure any disease or your money back. When you are taking their pills there is no guaranty of them curing anything, they always leave a loophole and of course there are side effects.

If a doctor says you have a disease that is incurable, get away from that doctor and find a better one. Any doctor who believes a disease is incurable is an ignorant person who doesn't deserve your time or attention. All diseases, every single one of them is curable, the difficulty is in finding the cure. You have to try one approach and if doesn't work, then you try another and another till you find the one that works.

You can be cured of any disease you have no matter if it is a chronic disease that you had for many years. Once you understand and accept this concept you have taken your first step toward curing it. No disease is 100% fatal, even the worst disease has a survival rate of about 5% percent. This meant that 5% of the people found a way to defeat the disease. If one-hundredth people get the disease it means that 5 people will survive it. You have to learn from those five survivors what they did to defeat their disease.

USES FOR MODERN MEDICINE

Some may think that I am totally against modern medicine, because of many of my writings and beliefs, but that is not totally true. I do believe that modern medicine actually can play a role in our health. Modern medicine has many defects, weaknesses and limitations, but it also has some strengths and those are the ones we need to learn so that we can properly use modern medicine.

The greatest strength of modern medicine is in traumatic injuries. If you have a broken arm, a deep cut or some other bodily injury then by all means go quickly to a modern doctor or hospital you need quick emergency modern medical attention. Diet, meditation or any other alternative medicine cannot heal any body injury, it just won't happen. In traumatic injuries modern medicine just can't be beat. If I break something, I know I can not heal it by taking some tea; I will just go to the hospital, get an x-ray and get a cast.

Another great strength of modern medicine is in its diagnostic capabilities. Most doctors are great at diagnosing what is wrong with a person, of course they might have problem recommending a good cure, but they are pretty good at telling you what is wrong with your body. So if you were sick I would strongly recommend going to a modern doctor and let the doctor use the modern tools of medicine to find out what is your problem. I would take the diagnoses of a doctor and have it confirmed by another doctor, and then accept it. No I will not argue with their diagnosis, I am sure they will get that part right.

A third great strength of modern medicine is in its surgical ability. It can replace a disease organ with a healthy one from a donor. It can also perform surgery on deformities and other problems of a similar kind. These are problems that only the knife of an expert surgeon can remedy; no amount of yoga or massage will seal an internal injury.

The problem with modern medicine is in its inability to understand and accept its limitations. Most doctors feel that if modern medicine does not have a drug or surgery that can cure a disease, then there is no cure for the disease. That is a shortsighted view that closes the door to other possible ways of dealing with a disease.

Although the greatest weakness of modern medicine is in its reliance of drugs for every disease, there are times when you should take these drugs. When the pain is so acute that you can hardly stand it then it is the correct time to take the analgesic or when the disease is in such an advanced stage that drastic measures have to be taken to stop the disease in its tracks then it is OK to take the drugs. In those kinds of emergencies dealing with the disease by any means necessary takes precedence over side effects or whatever; however these should be only the rare occasions.

I usually use natural medicine to heal myself, but I must confess that there have been times when the problem was serious enough, for those few times I have taken drugs, of course I was aware that after the emergency had passed, I would need to detoxify my body from the drugs.

Patients need to realize that the longer they are on medical drugs the more dependent they become on them. Once the medical crisis is over then the patient needs to find a permanent cure and discontinue taking expensive and dangerous drugs. Discontinuing taking the drugs might take some time; the body often will crave the drug, so it needs to be detoxified. If you continually need to take antibiotics, then you have not fixed the problem that gives you those infections. The goal of every patient should be to get rid of the disease not to manage it and enrich the pharmaceutical industry.

Modern medicine can be of great help if used wisely. I have no doubt that with time modern medicine will get better and eventually begin to use some less drastic means to control disease instead of relying mainly upon drugs and surgery, their two favorite tools. I am sure that there will come a future time when modern medicine will integrate good nutrition and a healthy lifestyle as valid treatments and also accept many of the alternative cures into its fold.

TOXINS EVERYWHERE

We have put toxins everywhere. There are toxins in the air, in the water, in the ground and just about in any place and any item you can think of. We have even managed to load up nature with toxins. Some fish are now so toxically loaded with mercury that people can not longer eat them. All the foods in our markets are tainted with toxins.

Some people say that nature already has some toxic substances that we should not worry so much about man made toxins. Yes it is true that some natural products have toxins in them, but they were never as dangerous as the man made toxins and also never at the levels that artificial toxins are dumped into nature.

Since we are surrounded with toxins what can we do? We can do many things. We can start by removing toxins from our near environment. We need to avoid using pesticides in our gardens and instead use natural means of pest control. We need to avoid using toxic cleaners in our house and resort to more natural cleaning substances. We need to quit using toxic deodorizers in our homes, carpets and pets.

Stop buying toxic products. Don't buy any toys that have lead paint in them. Don't buy ceramics with lead. Stop buying plastic kitchenware that leach carcinogens into your food, instead buy stainless steel, or some other safe material for your food.

We also need to stop loading our bodies with toxins by refusing to buy highly toxic deodorants, soaps and shampoos. We need to quit using toxic in our skin; this includes chemical sun tan lotions. We need to switch to natural products. If you wouldn't eat then you should not put in your skin. For whatever you put in our skin will eventually penetrate your body. Your skin is part of your body, if you put poison on your body; it is just as bad as if you were eating it.

We also need to detoxify our internal system. We need to detoxify our bodies, and cleanse ourselves from all the toxins that are accumulated over time. Some people will say that there is no need to detoxify our bodies because it is a new concept, which many of the ancients did not know about. The ancients did not have to detoxify their bodies, because they did not live in the toxic soup that we practically swim in every day.

There are many ways that people use to detoxify their systems. Some use an all organic cleanse, others use herbal teas and some use juices. Some people advice doing a water cleansing while others advice deep breathing exercises and some others advocate some other methods. Some methods may be more effective than others are, but the most important point is to do something, to take action in order to detoxify your body.

Which method of detoxification is the best? Every method has it champions, but the best method is the one that you can actually follow. The more demanding and complex the method the less likely that you will follow it. So it is not about which method is best, but which method you can actually follow. Of course if a method that you are following does not give you more energy and pep in your life, then you should try something different. You can also try a combination of detoxification methods to get better results.

AIR YOURSELF

Oxygen is life; we breathe it into our lungs to live; it cleanses our bodies and provides fuel. Air is very important to our bodies; it is used for many biological processes. But we have a big problem if we live in the city; our air is contaminated. The body has to work harder to extract the life giving oxygen from impure air.

We do have two nice air filters in our lungs. But unfortunately they were not made to handle the amount of pollution that is currently in the air. That is the reason why we have so many respiratory diseases. Seriously we can not breathe filth constantly and not get sick eventually.

The bigger or more enclosed a city is, the bigger the effects of the pollution. Pollution lingers longer in an enclosed city. And to make matters worse we continue to constantly add more and more pollution to the air. We have way too many cars, and factories spewing their poison into the air.

The air has a cycle process that cleanses any pollution in it, but it works on its own schedule not ours. The cycle of nature constantly removes some pollution from our cities, but we add more than what nature removes. Even if we stop adding a single bit of pollution to the air, it will take years for the polluted air to clear from the major cities.

What can you do about this health problem? You can do your part, you can make sure that your car does not pollute or better yet, do not have a car. You can walk, use a bike, share a ride or use public transportation. You can avoid using products that pollute the air, you can plant a few trees and of course you can apply political pressure for clean air.

Get away from the pollution; go to the great outdoors where there are plenty of trees, and fresh water. Go deep into the ocean, or at least go to the city parks. The whole point is to go to a place that has lots of clean fresh air. The top of a mountain is a perfect place to get some clean air and practice deep breathing exercises.

Learn to breathe deeply, practice some breathing exercises and inhale all the good oxygen from nature. I would recommend inhaling oxygen, but oxygen tanks are flammable and very dangerous. If you get a chance to get some clean oxygen then go for it. That is why exercise is important, it makes you breathe deeply and use your oxygen better.

If you have a ventilation system make sure it is working good and change the filter often. Some houses and buildings suffer from bad ventilation, the air is not properly circulated and pockets of polluted air get created. Open the windows and the doors once in a while and let the air come in and cleanse the place.

Smoking tobacco or marihuana will destroy your lungs. They are already stressed out dealing with pollution. If a co-worker smokes, then ask politely if he can not blow the smoke your way. It is your health and you have every right to protect it, just don't start a fight. Smoking is not a private vice; it is shared with all those people around the smoker.

WATER IS LIFE

Water is life without water there is no life. The main problem is that we have polluted our water. We need to make sure that you do not drink water that is contaminated or has harmful bacteria. Drinking water that is unhealthy is a cause of many diseases around the world. That is why you should never drink any water that you have no idea where it comes from. Purified drinkable water is the only water to drink.

Never, never, never drink water from the faucet. It is not healthy not matter what the water department says. The employees in the water department in Los Angeles actually had bottled water delivered to their main offices while at the same time they were telling people that their water was safe to drink. If they were not willing to drink their own water, it makes you wonder what they knew that the public doesn't. I strongly recommend getting water filters yes they are expensive, but the health benefits are great.

You probably have heard that you should drink 8 glasses of water per day, but the truth is that everyone is different and people have different needs for water. It depends on the diet that you eat; how active you are and your body type. The majority of the people live in a dehydrated state, which they attempt to remedy by using sugary or caffeinated drinks, which only makes the situation worse. For some people with health problems 8 glasses would not be enough. No drink can substitute for water, it is an irreplaceable substance, nothing can hydrate the body the way plain purified water does.

I would go so far as to advice people to avoid bathing in regular water. I strongly recommend buying a shower filter. Why? Because regular tap water has chlorine and other harmful chemicals and your skin absorbs everything that is upon it. Yes the skin has a marvelous defense mechanism, but any substance put on the skin will eventually penetrate your body. This is a well-known medical fact, which is the reason people wear chemical medical patches.

If you have health problems there is water healing. Water as medicine might strike some people as a new concept but it has been used for centuries in some cultures. The person drinks water to purify the body and bathes in pure water to cleanse the system. This is done for a few days. This water fast is a tremendous healer for many intestinal diseases. After two or three days of only drinking water the subject begins introducing soft foods that are easy in the stomach; usually vegetables and green herbs.

Some people believe in taking hot steam baths to open the skin pores and let the body toxins come out. Bathhouses are still popular in many countries. The Romans and other ancient cultures used to soak in hot water to treat many of their diseases. Natural hot springs are popular with natural healing advocates.

Water is good for you drink it, bath in it and soak in it. Plain purified water can actually heal some people from diseases. Water sustains and give life, but of course too much of a good thing can also be bad. Excessive drinking of water can actually cause a condition called water intoxication, in which a person will start acting like a drunk and can even die from it.

THE HEALING SUN

The modern idea that the sun is dangerous is plain wrong and foolish, it is erroneous and false propaganda. The sun is a powerful healing force. Sunlight gives life and vitality to this planet. The sun is good and gives energy; and you should take advantage of that free energy. To get the free power of the sun all you have to do is simply step outside and uncover your skin. Let the healing rays of the sun fall upon your body and get all its wonderful benefits. Sunlight is a magnificent tonic able to bring health and well being to your body.

The sun provides us with vitamin D and other health benefits. The sunlight that gives us warm is also an excellent way to block pain, disinfect wounds, heal the body and provide us with energy. Sunlight has been used in the treatment of tuberculosis, eczema, sleep disorders, Seasonal Affective Disorder

(SAD), and even in Multiple Sclerosis. Children not exposed enough to the sun can get a terrible disease called rickets and also asthma.

The big problem is that we modern people are not used to the power of the sun, we have spent most of our lives hiding from the sun under the mistaken notion that is bad for us. That is why we need to ease into using the healing power of the sun, we need to adjust our bodies to accept sunlight otherwise we will get sunburn. We have to start out with a 10-minute sun-bath every day for at least a couple of weeks and then increase the dosage little by little the amount of time till we can get at least one hour per day.

No, you will not get skin cancer from exposure to the sun; that is a myth. The biggest factors for getting skin cancer are a poor diet, bad habits and sun blockers. Yes believe it or not, but those sun blockers contain powerful carcinogenic chemicals that not only block the healing power of the sun, but actually cause cancer. People who live in the tropical regions do not develop skin cancer despite a life of prolonged exposure to the sun. According to modern beliefs; these people should be dropping like flies, yet few of them ever develop skin cancer.

If you eat a poor diet, if you smoke tobacco, or marijuana; if you drink a lot of coffee or other toxic substances you are in a toxic state. The sunlight helps the body expel those substances out of the body by the means of sweat and once those toxins are in your skin they can accumulate and cause skin cancer.

The sun actually prevents and heals skin cancer; it can also help with cancer in the breast, the ovaries, the colon and prostate cancers. Some health advocates believe that sunlight can help to protect against 16 types of cancer. It is those people who had the most exposure to the sun who suffer from the lowest incident of those types of cancers.

Of course our modern lifestyle has also affected our capacity to receive the full benefits of the sun. We have polluted the air and it has caused the sun to be obscured. That is why it is best to get away from the city, and got to a mountain or to the beach to get the full benefits of sunlight.

And don't worry about getting wrinkles or drying of the skin from sun exposure, those are myths too. Listen, and listen good you do not get wrinkles or dried skin from the sun, you get it from a poor diet, bad habits and even from those toxic skin lotions. Get over those silly notions that the life giving sun is dangerous to your health.

EARTHLING

We are people of the earth; we are made of the earth elements. We are earthlings; we sprang forth from the ground. In a sense the earth is our mother and we return to its fold on our death. We have forgotten this but we need to remember it if we want to continue living upon this earth.

Somehow in this new age we have lost touch with the fact that we are earthlings. We walk on carpet or linoleum covered floors. The sidewalks are made of hard concrete; the connection with the earth is being lost. We avoid the earth at all costs without realizing that we really need to get back in touch with the earth.

Farming is now done by less and less people, it seems that people are getting away from the earth and the further away from the earth we get, the sicker we get. Not only that; but we now pollute the good farming soil with chemicals and pesticides.

We now seem to think that there is something wrong with touching the ground from which we are made, that it is filthy. Yes the ground is polluted because of all the bad substances we pour upon it, but the ground without pollutants is good. Animals thrive in the ground and plants live in it. Clean and unpolluted ground is good and life giving.

If you go away from civilization get a hold of some good ground, smell it, feel it, taste it; yes I did say taste it. Good ground has plenty of minerals and plant debris in it that is how it gives life to plants and animals. You are made of the earth, you are an animal and the earth is good for you too. No I am not saying you should eat dirt for lunch, what I am saying is that we need to get over the idea that contact with the earth is somehow evil.

You need the minerals that the earth has; you also need salts and other nutrients that come from the ground. Of course you get these nutrients from the plants, but you can bypass the plant world and get minerals directly from the earth. No I repeat I am not advocating eating dirt, but to stop thinking that a little dirt is harmful. So what if your organic carrots have a little dirt on them, eating a little fertile nontoxic soil is not going to kill you, it actually might help you digest the food better.

Cleanliness is good but when carried to an extreme that all contact with the earth is avoided then it begins to affect our health and our life. Get on some clean ground and roll in it, go the ocean and roll in the beach. Walk barefooted in some mountain and feel the earth beneath you. Barefoot walking will massage your feet and reconnect you to the earth.

Some people advocate mud baths, and I agree that mud baths are a good therapy. Mud baths perform a double duty, the minerals and other substances in the good mud will penetrate your body and the mud will absorb the toxins from your body. You have to understand that not all mud is alike; there are certain places that have excellent mud full of good minerals that your body can absorb.

There are some people who advocate eating small doses of earth from certain places, because of the minerals and other healthful substances they contain. If you can be sure that the ground is not polluted or contains harmful bacteria and don't mind going for it, there is nothing wrong with putting a small teaspoon of this ground on your water and drinking it. No you will not die or get sick from eating a little teaspoon of mud.

The earth is your friend; it gave you life and continues to give you life through the plants that grow in it. The earth is vibrant and full of life. Cherish the good things that come from the earth. If you have a garden; then grow your own food and feed the soil with good compost.

THE BIGGEST ORGAN

The biggest organ in our body is the skin. This part of our body is the main protection our whole body has. This is the only organ that is exposed to the outside world and perhaps the most abused and vulnerable. It is your presentation wrapper; your skin is what people see of you.

The skin absorbs anything that is put into it and it carries it back into the body. That is why the nicotine patch is used to slowly release medicine into the body. That is why patches of x medicine are put into heart patients. Our biggest organ is absorbent while at the same time is protective.

The skin has antifungal and antibacterial properties; it has a layer of fat to keep us warm. It has fussy hairs that have sensory functions. It has also pores, and many other pieces. The skin is a wonder of engineering, able to do a multitude of functions.

It also has a porous system that expels toxins from the body to the outside world. Sweat is water mixed with salts and other toxic substances that the body has rejected. When a person smells badly it is because the top layer of skin is loaded with toxins and pollutants and needs to be cleansed. We need to shower in clean, non-chlorinated water.

Some people use deodorants to hide body odors instead of addressing the reason for those body odors. If a person constantly smells bad it is because of the toxic diet that person has. A bad diet will produce bad odors; it is as simple as that. Deodorants only hide the smell they do not get rid of the cause of the odors.

Antiperspirants are a modern invention and they are all bad. People who use antiperspirants do not seem to understand that they are going against nature. The body is made to sweat, that is what those glands are for. The moment you put on antiperspirants you are blocking the exits for the toxins in your body. Sweat is not your enemy; it is a healthy process that allows your body to get rid of excess salts and other toxic substances.

People who are healthy do not smell and they do not need to use antiperspirants or deodorants. If you want to smell nice then you can try some natural lotions. You can do like the ancients and anoint your body with olive oil and smelling spices. These contain no harmful cancer causing chemicals like the modern deodorants do.

Pamper your skin it deserves it after all it does for you. Take a mud bath or a steam bath in a natural spring. Go for a swim in a non-polluted place. Another great thing that you can to your skin is to massage it. Yes go have a nice body massage and let your body relax and feel great. Once in a while massage your feet, your hands and your legs.

Take care of your skin, it protects you, so you go ahead and protect it. Do no put on cancer producing products on your skin. There are plenty of natural alternatives for your skin. Give your body a rest from toxic products; get some natural soap for your body wash with natural made shampoo instead of those toxic shampoos and conditioners.

THE BITTER TRUTH

The bitter truth is that we humans are largely responsible for the poor health we may have. Our health really is in our hands and we are not doing a good job of keeping it. The many health problems that our modern society suffers from are basically self-inflicted. It is not that I am heartless, or want to be mean but if you have health problems it is because you brought them upon yourself. Yes I know that people do not want to hear this, but it is the truth; if you are sick it is mostly your fault.

We would like to blame our poor health on our genes, on some external force, but that is seldom the truth. No it is not the fault of your parents or your race if you have diabetes, high blood pressure, are obese or have some other disease. There are plenty of people who had both diabetic parents and they do not develop diabetes.

If you abuse your body with drugs, alcohol or tobacco, you have to pay the price eventually. When cancer comes upon you, you shouldn't be surprised; you are reaping exactly what you have sown. If you eat garbage, you will have all kinds of diseases, and no you can not blame it on your bad luck or reproach God.

If you are sick you may ask why, the answer is pretty simple, why not? Do you think you can mistreat and abuse your body and don't pay for it? Do you think you can drink all those poisonous sodas and don't get sick? Do you think you can eat like a pig and don't look like one? You can not violate the natural laws without paying the penalty.

So what can you do? Well you can stop. Yes that is the first step toward healing. You have to stop doing what caused the disease in the first place. If you have diabetes you have to stop eating sugar. If you have high blood pressure you have to stop abusing salt. If you have frequent stomach problems you simply have to stop eating badly.

Stop, stop, stop; this might sound like an easy step to take, but you may be surprised by how many people continue on abusing their bodies, despite their health problems. If you have acid reflux instead of taking an anti-acid medicine, why don't you simply stop eating what is causing your acid reflux.

There are plenty of people who have a heart problems or cancer, and have an operation to take care of that problem, but in a year or two they have the same problem again. They kept on eating those foods that caused the cholesterol or cancer.

The next step after stop is to start. You have to start doing the opposite of what was causing the disease. You have to start doing those things that are healthful, you have to start taking preventive steps, and you also have to start eating healthy.

We are killing ourselves yet we expect the doctors and surgeons to correct the problems that we have created. Sorry to tell you but there is not magical pill that will cure stupidity. It is up to you to take of your health by taking preventive steps, eating healthy and stop doing those things that are harmful to your body and mind. It is only when we accept personal responsibility that we can prevent disease or regain our health.

LIFESTYLE OF EXCESS

One of the reasons many people have poor health is because they have a lifestyle of excess. Let us face it many people have a lifestyle that never sets limits, their lifestyle of excess is hurting their health and killing them. If you lead a life of excess you will dissipate your energies and time, you will get sick and you will not enjoy life.

Many people lack restrain in what they do. They do not drink a cup of coffee in the morning and call it quits; they keep on pepping up throughout the day. One teaspoon of sugar isn't enough to sweeten their coffee; it has to be Half & Half (Half caffeine, Half sugar). One candy bar is not enough; they need to be chewing at all hours. They do not drink one soda from the machine and quit, no they must have soda after soda. At lunchtime they must get the triple burger and supersize their meals every time.

After work a single beer to relax is just not enough, they must have a six pack. If they smoke one cancer stick per day just won't do; they must be constantly puffing like a chimney. Watching a little TV is not possible, they must watch for hours on end. Playing videos games becomes a marathon. A small bag of snacks won't do, it must be the mega size bucket.

When they are invited or go out, they go all out. When they go to party a glass of wine is never enough; they have to get blasted. They do not dance a few times; no they must dance the night away. If they go to the beach they must sunbathe till they are well done. If they go to a restaurant it has to be an all you can eat type.

Restrain is not in their vocabulary and then they wonder why get afflicted with all kinds of diseases. They are just reaping what they have sown. The multitude of diseases plaguing our modern society is well earned. As a society we do not practice moderation in what we do, and then we wonder about the results.

Some people eat fried and greasy foods like there is no tomorrow and then complain about getting fat, and having heart attacks. They eat sugar by the pounds and then wonder why they get diabetes. They eat all their snacks salty and then wonder why they have high blood pressure. Come on people, the only reason they don't drop like flies, is because their bodies can withstand a lot of abuse.

These types of people live in denial; they refuse to believe that they do things excessively. Even when shown that they do, they try to excuse or minimize their excesses. Some say that they only drink on weekends, maybe that is true or not, but what is certain is that in the weekend they drink enough to make up for the whole week. It might have been less harmful if they had distributed their drinks throughout the week. At least their bodies might have a chance to handle it.

An excessive lifestyle will destroy your health and kill you. Some may balk and say that they must have some joy in life, that I am just a killjoy. Telling people to have some restraint is not being a killjoy or wet blanket. I am not opposed to having fun, but everything must be done in moderation. Of course this does not mean using hard drugs, marihuana or anything harmful in moderation, no sane person advocates that.

MY RESPONSE TO CRITICS

Some people will question my motives for disparaging the Big Food and Big Pharma corporations and heaping praise on the health food and botanical stores. First of all, I do not own a health food or botanical store; I make zero money from promoting healthy food or natural herbs. I do not get money for promoting bananas, apples and oranges. I get zilch for praising lettuce and cabbage. Nobody pays me anything, no organic farmer pays one red penny and no herbalist gives me a plug nickel.

The only reason I speak against the big corporations is because that they are simply selling us junk. Yes that is the truth. I am sure that there are plenty of good people working at those foods corporations and pharmaceutical companies; I am not saying they are evil, I can not judge people's motives, for all I can judge is their products. And with all due respect for their feelings, I will simply say that their products are hurting and killing us, a pretty simple truth, but one that sends some of them into a frenzy rage.

Why are they selling us those bad products, it is not really out of malice but out of a desire to make the most profit for their companies. The food manufacturers loose billions of dollars in spoilage, so they use chemicals that prevent that; unfortunately those chemicals are poison to human beings. Another way to keep food from spoiling is by processing it, but the process they use to preserve food, actually destroy nutrients and leave us with worthless food.

The pharmaceutical companies are also big business and they too must find ways to increase their profits. They are in the business of selling drugs; they are basically drug pushers. Sure some of their drugs take away the symptoms of a disease and might make people feel better, but unfortunately in the long run most of their drugs are harmful. Those drugs often only mask the disease; they do not take care of the root cause of the disease and sometimes those drugs actually make the disease even worse, and I have not even begun to mention that most of those drugs produce so many side effects, that it might be better just living with the disease.

It is pointless to try to convince the store manager to quit selling us junk, the store manager has zero power to make any product changes. The only ones that have power to make changes are the executives. But they too are reluctant to make any changes that will hurt the bottom line. You see the food and pharmaceutical executives are under the gun to produce profits or lose their jobs, so they do everything that is legal and in their power to make those profits. I am sure most of those executives do not want to hurt people, but the system is rigged against the best interest of the consumer.

It is a good thing that my livelihood does not depend on the food or pharma industry, for then I could never speak against what they are doing to us. Some will say that I am not a doctor or a nutritionist, I consider that a plus in my favor, for that means that I have no vested financial interest in what I am teaching. If people listen to me, I make absolutely no monetary gain, so I do not have to worry about offending anyone. I am not going to lose or gain any money because of what I teach.

I make zero, zilch, nada money whether you follow or disregard my teachings. I am simply a voice crying out in the wilderness; warning people about the dangers in our current practices and teaching people about healthy living.

To my many current and future critics, I tell them to simple write to me and tell me precisely where I am wrong, so far I have not made any major corrections or recantations of anything that I have written. Please refrain from writing to me with insults and ignorant comments; I am not going to bother to even read those. I prefer to spend my time reading about those things that will benefit my health.

Listen, friends you might hear those critics speaking evil about me and my ideas, well I am not that interested in defending my reputation, I am more interest in helping people achieve health. I do not have time to waste dealing with the critics.

IT IS YOUR DECISION

The old saying that "you can lead a horse to the water, but can not make him drink" is quite true. In here, I have written plenty of ideas and suggestions on how to keep and improve your health, but accepting them and acting on them it's your decision. No one is going to go and check up on you.

If you secretly are doing illegal drugs, you will eventually be found out. Don't fool yourself into thinking that you can control them, you can not. One day you will lose control and your world will come crashing down. The penalties are severe not only in your health, and your money, but you will probably lose your job and even your freedom.

If you have bad health habits you can continue on them if you want to. You can continue living a life style of excess; smoking, drinking and partying late into the night and then going to work in the morning and perking up with buckets of coffee. Plenty of people do it. However think that what you eat or drink will affect your body and your mind. And how you feel and think will affect your job performance.

You can continue eating all that garbage from the supermarket, getting your fill of sugar, fat, salt, and white flour. No one is going to check your grocery list. However don't go crying and complaining when you develop horrible diseases from your nutrition. Well you can cry and complain, but it will do you little good.

If you do not exercise do not expect to have a healthy body; that is just not going to happen. You can try buying all those magical pills, creams, wraps and other gadgets advertised on TV, but you are just wasting your money. There is no shortcut to getting in shape; muscles are only created through exercise, simple as that.

You can continue ignoring the invisible killers of germs & radiation and refuse to clean up yourself, your house or your workplace; you can also continue to indulge in your electronic lust without restrain and continue nuking your food with the microwave. You can ignore these things, but ignoring their effects will not make them go away.

If you do not practice safety and security; you are bound to have problems. There is no safety and security unless someone bothers to implement them. If something happens and you get hurt, you can call the police or file a lawsuit, but they can not restore your health, providing of course that you survive the accident or attack.

Your emotions and reactions are your own; no one can make you angry, afraid or nervous unless you allow them. No one can stress you out unless you allow him or her. Your mental state is under your complete control. But if you have an altered mind by eating harmful substances you really have lost control.

You can keep on hoping for that magical pill that will cure all diseases and ills, but there is none. You can believe the lies of the pharmaceutical companies and take their deadly drugs, but don't expect healing from them. The sooner you accept this reality the sooner you can take control of your health. You are responsible for the lifestyle you lead.

PREVENTION

The best way to be healthy is to keep it that way. Of course there are some individuals who were born with health problems or developed them early in life. However the majority of people manage to reach adulthood in reasonable good health.

When people are young and healthy they tend to think that it will always be that way. But if they do not take care of themselves, they will in time learn the hard way that good health needs to be protected. Many people deeply regret the lifestyle they have led and wish they could turn the clock back and start over, but it is just not possible.

If you do not suffer from any disease then you need to keep yourself that way. You need to take precautions and avoid doing those things that could negatively affect your health. You need to learn and develop the habits that will keep you healthy for the rest of your life. Your body is not indestructible; it will eventually show the abuse you have given it.

Can you prevent disease, yes you can. Listen we live in an ocean of bacteria, yet most of us manage to remain healthy. It is those individuals who have not taken care of themselves that usually end up with all the diseases. There are some senior citizens that are in better health than most middle-aged people are. And not it is not because those seniors have good genes; it is because those seniors took good care of their bodies in their youth.

What are some of the things you can do to keep healthy? Well you can eat properly and follow a healthy lifestyle. You can take proper care of you body, by showering, washing your hands whenever needed and brushing your teeth and sleeping properly. You can do schedule some regular exercise daily. There are many things that you can do to prevent disease and keep healthy.

Another important step is to have yearly checkups. Have blood test done and a complete physical once or twice per year. The earlier a disease is caught the easiest it is to treat it. Once you allow a disease to grow, it sometimes become impossible to get rid of it.

Disease is expensive, very expensive. Not only in terms of money but also in terms of quality of life. Disease will also take a lot of your time and fun in life. Disease becomes an impediment or obstacle that you have to deal with every day. Once your body develops a chronic disease it is usually there to stay. And even if the disease is cured there will be residual effects that might last a lifetime.

Prevention is the cheapest medicine around and it is a life prolonger. By the time most people reach their middle age their bodies have been neglected for so long that they just simply start giving up. There are millions of people who take better care of their cars or their lawns than their bodies.

No I am not advocating that you become a total health fanatic and spend every minute of your life obsessing about your health, but you do have to practice a little preventive maintenance of your body and mind, every day.

****

NOTE FROM THE AUTHOR

I hope you have enjoyed these few words that I have written. I am still in the process of doing more research in the field of natural health, for I find it a fascinating and useful field

I am not a famous person; that you should listen to me; all I have done is to deeply study these areas for they were of interest to me. And I decided to share my findings with others so that they perhaps will find something in here that might alleviate their suffering.

Thru the years I have accumulated many notes on different areas of natural health, I would like to develop some of those into book length and publish them for the benefit of those interested in natural healing.

Please write me or e-mail me to let me know what fields you will like to know more about, so that I can do more research in those areas and give you readers the most valuable information I can find from different sources.

I have no notions of being a great teacher or a wise sage, all that I am is a person who found healing in nature and I want to share with others some of the steps I took to find my own healing.

A simple voice crying out in the wilderness